THE EDGE OF THE SCALPEL

By the same author

The Transforming Knife
The Secret Knife
The Healing Knife
Crusader's Clinic
The Years of the Healing Knife

THE EDGE OF THE SCALPEL

GEORGE SAVA

WILLIAM KIMBER · LONDON

First published in 1983
WILLIAM KIMBER & CO. LIMITED
100 Jermyn Street
London SW1Y 6EE

ISBN 0-7183-0469-1

Photoset in North Wales by
Derek Doyle & Associates, Mold, Clwyd
Printed in Great Britain by
Biddles Limited, Guildford and Kings Lynn

Contents

Prologue

They all come to your consulting room or to the hospital out-patients' department with one thought uppermost in their minds: the fervent hope that you may be the man to help them.

You know little or nothing about them. They are just names in the appointments' book. Someone speaks to you on the telephone; another desperate search for help.

You return from lunch and your secretary or the hospital nurse tells you that Mr Smith or Miss Brown is coming to see you at two o'clock the next day. The nurse enquires politely if it will be convenient for the patient to come directly to the hospital.

It is your first free afternoon that week and you had hoped to have a well-deserved rest ... But no matter – another human being is seeking your help. Yet the name you have just jotted down in your diary might as well be that of the paramount Chief of some Melanesian Island as that of an Australian land-owner or staid-looking Mrs Helen Jones.

It is just a name, an entry, a time, a date ... until you meet.

Miss Brown may have been a devastating beauty once; that middle-aged man has come to the end of his tether. The sallow woman may be suffering from some rare and dangerous illness, making her dear to the eye of the surgeon and raw material for a possible paper in the medical journals – or she may be just one more rich hyponchondriac. She may even be one of those remarkable people who think they ought to have an operation in order to have a riveting conversation piece at a far from riveting party.

Their illnesses and disorders may be different but many of them share one thing: they have not responded to conventional medical and surgical treatment. Therefore they are prepared to take risks.

There is a knock at your door and a name placed before you. A little later, the patient arrives. The name has become a person – very often a frightened or desperate one – certainly one ill at ease.

It may be a self-confident man with a healthy contempt for doctors, who, he impresses upon you, have not been able to help him. Or it may be a reticent young woman who is under the impression that doctors and surgeons are a race of supermen set above other mortals and can bring about the impossible at the touch of a wand.

Little by little, you absorb stories. You may be their last hope after they have received refusal after refusal from other surgeons, or after they have tried countless remedies and costly concoctions – all to no avail.

Your name may be pronounced in ecstasy or barked at you as if it were that of an evil-doer. You may not even be called by a name at all, but merely addressed by that respectable and respectful label of 'Doctor'.

Yes, they are little more than walking names, fresh cases to whom the same routine of questions has to be put, for whom a new card has to be filled in for the index. They have signs and symptoms – some of them. They may be in search of something other doctors have been unable to supply. They may be fighting hard and resolutely for a life that is slipping from them.

But for you they are still no more than cases and types. You have met the person who argues that your diagnosis is as wrong as the one he received from the last physician he consulted. Oh, how often you have met him! You know equally well the one who is prepared to try anything – no matter what and no matter how unpleasant – just to receive some relief from his agonising malady.

Little by little something of their personality emerges. They cease to be names and gradually, they assume individuality, with their secret fears and hopes, their hidden joys and sorrows. They are people, after all – people of flesh and blood; very often suffering flesh and blood which it is up to you to mend! And step by step you try to win their confidence, and for a time being you and the patient become parts of a team working for one end – the patient's health and happiness.

They lose their reserve and tell you more about themselves, something more than medical histories can and you dip deep into the infinite variety of the human soul. It is then that the final metamorphosis has been made. No longer are they names or case-histories. They are real people who will survive in your memory. They tell stories of tragedy and stories of fulfilment, and each is different from the other ... Different yes – still they have one thing in common – they have been declared inoperable, incurable by accepted remedies; or they are simply terminal.

And it is here that your own impotence and despair grips you. You listen to their stories and you know deep down in your heart that you cannot help in any way. Everything that you have learnt and been trained to do has been tried without success.

You have heard of unorthodox methods – faithhealing, hypnosis, acupuncture, herbal concoctions. But you are not allowed to use them. They are methods not recognised by the medical orthodox fraternity. You have taken the Hippocratic Oath to help suffering humanity. It does not instruct you on how to do it or what remedies to adopt. That is left to your own judgement and experience. Have you the right to disregard all the canons of orthodox medicine? If you do, you might be accused by some of your colleagues as an irresponsible surgeon. You certainly cannot disregard their opinion. Then you ask yourself:

'Have I the right to deny any remedy, no matter how unorthodox and unpopular, to the man or woman who is sitting before me and in whose eyes one can discern the trembling hope or dread that you too will tell them they are beyond help.'

It is some of these very stories that I have set down in the following pages. They are medical stories – yes; but they are not mere case histories. They are stories of men, women and children who have come to the last gateway of release from this or that sickness. Each gave me a new glimpse of the baffling thing we call Life. Each was a living proof that there are no two people exactly alike in the whole universe.

Could I deprive them of that last hope?

'No,' I decided. 'I'll try any remedy, adopt any surgical procedure as long as I am satisfied that if it will not help, at least it will not harm either.' To some I explained that the remedy was not recognized by orthodox medicine; to others that the surgical technique might even be dangerous in their state of health. They spoke the same words as if from one mouth. 'I have nothing to lose, Doctor!'

In thinking back, I have done many things of which I could perhaps be sincerely proud and things that gave me great satisfaction. Granted, perhaps, in some cases I also did things I should not have done – performing operations that entailed too many risks and were against the accepted rules and practices of orthodox medicine and surgery. But that did not mean that I performed unnecessary or risky operations. Risky yes, from my point of view, but not unnecessary. The patients all benefited from them.

'You were lucky to get away with it,' some friends would say after an operation that although very risky, had saved or prolonged a patient's life.

'Don't do it again, George!' cautious friends would warn. 'Even your luck cannot last for ever.'

That might be so, but I knew that without that 'risky' operation the patient might have died earlier. 'Conscience', said Hamlet, 'doth make cowards of us all'. How true that is, most of us know, often to our shame. But does not conscience also sometimes make brave men and women of us, inspiring us with unaccustomed courage and resolve to carry out things that, but for that still, small voice, would have remained undone?

In my work, conscience has always been my guide. At times it tormented me with doubts, accusations and promptings. Yes, there have been cases which involved an appeal to my conscience and intuition, to what today we call 'hunch'. No doubt in some instances I have broken conventions in one way or another, but in none have I *broken* the law, either of the land, or of my profession. So I have occasion for neither guilt nor shame.

'Thou shalt not admit that thou knowest not what to do.' Of that I was never guilty. I always knew what I was going to do. Sometimes risky to myself but never – in the final end – to the health and wellbeing of the patient.

These histories of patients I have treated by 'unorthodox' methods, and the results thereof are my defence.

I

Acupuncture Against Asthma

It is impossible to describe the agonies I endured, following my car accident. For six months I was practically confined to my home after the initial two days in the hospital to which the ambulance had taken me. I could scarcely move, nor could I sleep in a bed.

The only way I could get some rest was to sit in an armchair propped up with cushions and with my neck bandaged in a plaster of Paris cast. At times I wished I were dead. But somehow life asserted itself. I am not a religious man, but I could not help feeling that God did not wish me to join my departed parents and brothers yet. I had the strange sensation that my end was still a long way off.

And so the months dragged on. Slowly my strength returned. The pain began to recede gradually and I could get some rest without any pain-killing drugs.

Christmas was approaching. The year that had begun so promisingly was about to come to a close.

Did I have any future? At times I was still little more than an invalid, uncertain whether I would ever again hold a scalpel.

I was never one for sitting around and twiddling my thumbs. And I was not even now resigned to a life of uselessness and idleness. Those closest to me know and understand this.

So after spending a quiet Christmas I knew that for the time being I had to leave England once again. Subconsciously I felt that it would help me get over the shock psychologically. But where to? Australia!

Almost dreamlike the idea settled in my mind. True, my reception there had not been all it might have been that first time. Nevertheless, deep down I had developed a genuine fondness and love for the country and its people.

I flew to Perth, the capital of Western Australia. It was New Year's Eve. The plane touched down at five o'clock in the afternoon. I took a taxi and drove to the hotel I had booked from the Airport.

Six o'clock. Streets crowded with revellers determined to see the old year out and welcome the New Year in. I, alone of all those people, was not to join in, it seemed. Alone in the terrifying, unfriendly room of an impersonal hotel. Not an ideal way in which to spend New Year's Eve! Then an inspiration:

I would ring up a friend of mine. A doctor who had been one of the few ready to help me on that previous occasion. I found his name in the telephone-book and dialled the number. A friendly female voice answered.

'Who is this?' she wanted to know.

'A friend from London. Is Dr Miller available?'

Dr Miller was available and he recalled my name at once. 'Where are you, Dr Sava?' he asked excitedly. I gave him the name of the hotel.

'What are you doing this evening?'

'Nothing,' I admitted. 'I've only just arrived and I suppose bed is the best place for me.'

'Oh, no, it's not!' he laughed. 'You just stay where you are – we'll come and pick you up.'

'Pick me up? What for?'

'We're going to a friend's party – and you're jolly well coming with us!'

'Oh, I couldn't. I don't know these people. How can I descend on them – a total stranger. No, no – thanks. I just couldn't.'

'But we are not strangers and a friend of ours is a friend of his. The friend who is giving the party is a great man and a very good friend. That's quite sufficient,' insisted the generous Dr Miller. 'So no more arguments. We're coming for you.'

And so my friend and his lovely wife would not take no for an answer. In less than half an hour they were at the hotel and we renewed our old acquaintance.

The party was fabulous. One of those parties only a man of unlimited means and generous heart could give. We arrived just as dinner was being served. The host and hostess greeted my friend warmly. I was introduced. I began to apologise for the intrusion. Max Nardini, the host, soon put a stop to that.

'A friend of Dr Miller is a friend of ours. You are more than welcome, Dr Sava.' His charming wife smiled and nodded approvingly.

And that was just how I was made to feel from the beginning to the end. When I took my place at the dinner table I knew I was no intruder. These wonderful people made me feel infinitely at ease.

While we sipped brandy after dinner and waited to pop the champagne to welcome the New Year, Max Nardini asked me where I was staying. I told him the name of the hotel.

'Not too good,' was his comment.

'The only one I could get for to-night,' I explained. 'I simply couldn't get into a better one, everything was full up.'

'Well, you've got a better one now,' my host said nonchalantly.

'What d'you mean?'

'Just what I say,' he smiled. 'You've found a better place. You're coming to stay with us. We have room – and to spare!'

'But ...' I was flabbergasted. 'I couldn't surely! How can I impose on you like that?'

'You won't be imposing. We'd like you to stay. There is a vacant suite on the upper floor of our apartment. We think you'll like it. Right, Sandy?' He turned smiling to his wife.

'Of course, Dr Sava. Please come. We'll send for your luggage.' Her face radiated warmth and genuine friendliness. I felt too, that my loneliness was now a thing of the past.

I stayed for dinner. And I stayed on. A great many weeks had passed since that first momentous dinner and the ensuing New Year's Eve celebrations. At this stage I felt more like a member of the Nardini family. Even their two delightful children welcomed me in the way only children can, I became their 'Uncle' George, and their voices gladdened my lonely heart each time they spoke to me.

Professionally too, Australia seemed bent on making up to

me for its former negligence. I received my new registration with the Medical Board immediately. My doctor friend found me two patients who wanted plastic corrections.

I told him of my dreadful accident and what the doctors' verdict had been.

'Nonsense,' said Dr Miller. 'How do you know that you can't work if you don't try?' He eyed me challengingly: 'Operate!'

And I did. But before my first operation, I had to venture into a new, controversial field – acupuncture.

My host had many friends, both business associates and social. Stan Irlington was one of them.

He was a tall, handsome man in his early sixties, wealthy, and owner of vast lands in the fertile part of Western Australia. It was a casual talk with Max that brought Stan's name up in the conversation.

'Poor Stan,' my host was saying. 'He's terribly upset and dejected. All this land that produces the best apples in the whole of Australia. And now he has to sell everything!'

'Why?' I asked perplexed. 'Why should a man like Stan, who hasn't even reached retirement age have to do that? Why on earth should he sell land that is so productive?'

'Yes,' Max nodded. 'Stan loved that land and he says that life's not worth living without his living it on that land, growing and tending it.'

More puzzled than ever, I asked again: 'But why is he selling then?'

My friend looked sadly at me. 'It's his health. In the last two years Stan has developed some kind of allergy. He can't come near the orchards and the moment he begins work on the land, he gets terrible attacks of asthma which almost invariably land him in hospital.'

I wanted to hear more. My professional curiosity was getting the better of me. I asked for more information and Max suggested we went to visit Stan Irlington in his house.

We were received with open arms, both by Stan and his wife. I had to listen to an incredibly sad story.

Apparently, for no conceivable reason, the man developed severe asthma while staying on the land. He sought help from various doctors and specialists with no avail. Every kind of treatment was adopted and he would usually get better. The asthma would subside while he lived in the city, away from his estate. He would then feel well enough to attempt to get back to the land. And every time he would then end up back in hospital and eventually at his house in the city.

'It is like a prison for me,' he explained. 'I have no alternative but to sell everything and live in the city permanently.'

'It is a pity,' I commiserated. 'What do the doctors say? You have seen some specialists, no doubt?'

'Yes, I have seen the best in the country. But all they can say is that I have some kind of allergy to the dust or pollen. And that if I value my life – I must stay away from the land.' He paused for a moment. 'I have to sell. But what will I do in the city for heaven's sake?' he asked me imploringly as if I had the answer.

'You'll find something,' my host tried to console him. 'With all your experience, many companies will be only too pleased to have you on their boards as an executive.'

'Yes. But it will not be the same. I'll miss the land and orchards as long as I live.'

For a long moment I studied the miserable man. Suddenly, for no apparent reason my mind went back a few months, to when I witnessed a lecture by a doctor in London who had become an exponent of the ancient Chinese craft – acupuncture.

He was telling the audience how he had cured patients who did not respond to ordinary medical treatment.

I remembered that he mentioned asthma as one of the diseases that responded particularly well to acupuncture. I began to wonder. Had I the right to suggest something in which I myself did not wholly believe? Had I the right to give the man hope that might so easily turn to nothing?

My contact with the art of acupuncture had come quite by chance. I happened to receive an invitation to attend a conference on acupuncture held at the house of a London specialist.

There were several doctors attending and I was one of them, still all to sceptical of the new, unorthodox method. I say new – for me – but the art of acupuncture, of course, is the ancient Chinese method of both diagnosis and treatment of disease.

The name is not a Chinese one. In China itself the practitioners of this art seldom, if ever, called it by this name. For the Chinese doctors and people alike, the method is part of their philosophy of life on health and sickness.

Acupuncture has been known and practised for thousands of years in China and elsewhere in the Orient. This art of healing was given its name during the 17th Century AD by the Jesuit Fathers who were visiting Peking on a scientific mission.

Seeing how the Chinese doctors pricked their patients with silver and gold needles they named it acupuncture – a combination of the Latin words *acus* – needle – and *puncture* – puncture.

My next contact with acupuncture treatment came not by chance but by design. I wonder, had I known what adventures would befall me following my decision to study acupuncture, if I would have ventured at all.

This time it was Boston where I again came in contact with that ancient Chinese healing art.

After my curiosity had been aroused by the English acupuncturist's lecture and demonstrations, I agreed to attend the conference in Boston. It was given by the newly-formed International Institute of Acupuncture.

I took an active part in the debate that followed the lecture. I told them of what I had seen in London and to my surprise it must have impressed the director of the Institute.

After the lecture he invited me to dinner at his home. Later on, he asked me whether I spoke German. To my positive answer he smiled and said that he hoped I would do him and the institute a favour.

'What kind of favour?' I asked, puzzled. And you can imagine my surprise and certainly my delight when I learnt that he was willing to sponsor my trip to Vienna and enrol me at the clinic of Professor Johannes Bischko.

The man was the head of the only acupuncture clinic in Europe where he gave courses of three months for medical graduates. The doctor himself was one of the foremost exponents of the art of acupuncture in Europe and his courses were always attended by physicians from all over the world.

'We want you to go to Vienna and study with Professor Bischko,' the director told me. 'Then, we would like you to come back to Boston and organise our new institute. 'He looked at me poignantly: 'Will you do it?'

I could hardly believe my ears. I had already decided, even prior my visit to Boston, to learn more about acupuncture. And now I was given not only the chance to do that, but to study with the most famous acupuncturist in Europe. And what was more, even to be paid for the privilege. I accepted without any hesitation. The only thing I needed to know was how long they expected me to remain in Boston after the course in Vienna came to an end.

'As long as you wish,' the director replied. 'As a matter of fact, you can remain as the head of the institute. I believe you have American degrees so you can be registered as a medical practitioner in the State of Massachusetts.'

I explained that essentially my training was surgical and plastic surgery in particular, but that I was curious about acupuncture and would agree to remain for as long as it was necessary to train one of his own doctors.

The director agreed and before leaving his pleasant company, he handed me an envelope with a $500.00 cheque in it. 'If that is not enough, and you have to stay longer in Vienna, please wire us and I'll see that you receive an additional sum.'

That was more than generous at the time. I left the next morning for London and wrote immediately to Professor Johannes Bischko. The reply came in the form of a formal invitation and enrolment at the clinic to attend sessions on acupuncture.

What I saw and learned made me a convert. Admittedly, that a pinprick somewhere on the surface of the human body, more often than not away from the location of the illness or area of pain, should be able to cure or at least alleviate pain is almost impossible to credit, let alone to comprehend.

Doctors like myself, even when confronted with the evidence of patients who have been cured by acupuncture where other orthodox methods of treatment have failed, still somehow refuse to accept it as proven evidence. Yet it was there for everyone to see, to acknowledge as fact, even if not as a scientific experiment.

At the time the Jesuit Fathers christened the Chinese technique 'acupuncture', China was ruled by the Ming Dynasty and acupuncture was at its zenith.

There is no scientific explanation as to why it works, but work it does.

According to the Chinese philosophy of life, there are no diseases but diseased people and therefore every individual must be treated individually and often differently from others who might be suffering from the same disease.

All morbid conditions affecting human beings and animals for that matter are due to an imbalance of the vital forces of energy within the living creatures. This vital energy called in Chinese *Tsri* is expressed in dual form. *Yang* and *Yin* – the balance of those two forces constitutes the energy through which all living creatures flourish. The imbalance of *Yang* and *Yin* gives the diseases their particular symptoms and characteristics. Puncturing the skin with needles at well-defined points throughout the surface of the body, brings the two vital forces into balance again thus restoring the health of the individual.

For every disease or painful organ there are points where the needles must be inserted. These points are known and the needles have to be inserted along lines known as Meridians. There are however, a few reservations that have to be observed.

The first and most important reservation is that acupuncture must not be and cannot ever be a substitute for orthodox medicine and surgery. It can never substitute for a vital operation or for a life-saving drug. But if used as a helpful addition to the accepted surgical procedures or to the usual medications, it can become a really vital and important method of healing.

The other reservation is that acupuncture must only be practised by medically qualified doctors. If a quack, who by learning a few rules on acupuncture and a few vital points on insertion of needles along the Meridians of the human body, considers himself qualified to undertake to treat patients – he will only bring acupuncture into disrepute and cause nothing but sorrow or worse to his patients.

With these two reservations I can now define the fields of medicine and surgery where acupuncture can be of great service and immense help.

In surgery: not as a substitute but as an added help in alleviating the pains and discomforts that follow every operation. As post-operative pain-killers a few needles well placed at appropriate points along the corresponding Meridians can substitute almost entirely for sedative drugs and make the post-operative recovery painless and far speedier.

In medicine: In cases where chronic, intractable and painful conditions do not respond to accepted medication, acupuncture can be of inestimable help both to patients and medical practitioners.

In anaesthesia: Medical men the world over know that some patients are dangerously allergic even to the most proven anaesthetics. Some patients on the other hand, because of debilitating conditions, cannot tolerate either general or local anaesthesia. These can be helped by acupuncture used as a substitute for general or local anaesthesia.

Finally, acupuncture, well-administered, can be of help to elucidate some obscure symptoms thus helping to determine and arrive at a proper diagnosis.

These are the main fields of medicine and surgery where acupuncture in the hands of well-qualified men can be of vital help. It does not greatly matter that we don't know exactly why acupuncture works. There are no scientific bases to explain it and that's why it is called an art and not a science. The important thing is that it does help in many cases. Even in those cases where it cannot help it does not harm at least. For how many orthodox medical methods can we claim the same?

All this and more I learned at the clinic in Vienna from the brilliant lectures and demonstrations given by Professor Johannes Bischko. As I already had some knowledge of acupuncture, the Professor thought that I did not require the whole three months' training. Six weeks would be sufficient.

I tried to learn as much as I could and every week, I telephoned to the director in Boston telling him of my progress.

Soon my stay in Vienna was nearing its end, but an unexpected event was once again to change my plans.

I made friends with all the staff at the clinic and in the course of many conversations I told them about the new institute in Boston that I was supposed to organise. I told them that I did not think my six weeks' training was quite sufficient for the work required of me there.

At this point one of Bischko's assistants said that his one dream was to go to America, even for a short time. An idea struck me. I had learned all I needed about acupuncture but I was essentially a surgeon and the idea of spending my time as an acupuncturist without surgery did not appeal to me. I asked the young doctor if he would like to take my place in Boston. I pointed out to him that he was far more qualified to organise the institute than I.

He accepted eagerly. That very evening I spoke on the telephone with the director in Boston and explained the position. I told him that one of the assistants of Professor Bischko was willing to come to Boston and work as long as necessary for the institute. I said in all sincerity that he was far more qualified for the post than I could ever be.

The director assured me, that although he deeply regretted that our association could not come to fruition, he was deeply grateful to me for having found so well-qualified a doctor willing to come to Boston and organise the institute. I even received an invitation to visit them in the future whenever I came to Boston.

All I could do was thank him with all my heart and marvel again at American generosity, for he had insisted that the monetary grant they had given me and which I had offered to return, had been more than well-spent.

That settled it in the best possible way for all the parties concerned. I was preparing to return to London, when again destiny intervened.

Among the doctors attending the course I met two Israelis who were also learning acupuncture in addition to their training as surgeons. We became friends and one evening I went to bid them goodbye. They were sorry to see me go and one of them suggested that I come to Israel and stay with him for a few days. They were so utterly sincere in their wish for me to visit their country.

'You will like our country,' both of them enthused.

I admitted to having for a long time yearned to visit that ancient land where so much of the world's history had occurred.

'Then this is your chance!' beamed Dr Shatil. 'Why wait a moment longer?'

And not for the first time in my life, nor the last, I am sure, I yielded to impulse.

We, all three of us, received our certificates for the complete course in acupuncture and boarded the train from Vienna to Rome. The following day we flew El Al to Tel Aviv.

With great excitement I was anticipating the short, unexpected trip. I knew somehow that it would prove unique and unforgettable. How unique and unforgettable I was soon to discover. But it was certainly not what I had anticipated.

The plane touched down at five o'clock in the afternoon. It was a glorious, sunny afternoon. The air was heavy with heat. My dreams were of the exciting few days of sight-seeing, visiting the ancient landmarks – Jerusalem, Massada, Bethlehem, Nazareth, Tiberias – and all the other numerous historical places that have forever been part of the land of milk and honey.

The day was Friday – and at sundown, all shops closed. My friends explained it was the beginning of the Sabbath – but more – it was the eve of Yom Kippur – the 'Day of Atonement' – the most holy day in the entire Jewish year.

'We will rest at home,' my friend Yzchak told me. His wife waited for us, having driven to the airport in an old Morris Minor.

He introduced me to her, having previously phoned her

from Vienna to prepare her for my arrival.

She smiled a sweet smile of welcome, as if I were a long-lost friend. They both spoke fluent English and German, but we kept to English.

That evening, I witnessed the Sabbath blessing of religious people. Yzchak and his wife were sharing the house with his in-laws. The elderly couple, obviously very orthodox, stuck strictly to all the ancient laws of the Sabbath Eve. The old lady blessed the *chaleh* and then after she had lit the candles and said her prayers over them, I was handed a beaker from which we all sipped the sweet, ruby-red Israeli wine.

We talked until late in the night and then my friend showed me to my comfortable bedroom and bade me good-night. I must have slept heavily as I was rather tired and could not have heard the great upheaval in the early morning.

Still half asleep, I heard a knock on the door followed instantly by the entry of my friend. I could tell by his face that something was terribly wrong.

'What's the matter, Yzchak?' I asked. 'What's happened?'

'War has broken out!' he said.

'War? Overnight?' I could not believe my ears.

'Egypt and Syria have attacked us once again,' Yzchak said fatalistically, his face white and drawn. 'And on Yom Kippur, of all days, our most sacred day in the entire Jewish Calendar!'

'My God!' was all I could say.

'I've to report to my unit immediately, George. I'm a military surgeon and my duty is to be with the regiment.' After a short pause he added, 'I'm really sorry that your holiday is ruined. If I were you I would leave on the next plane. Our wars are no picnics!'

'I suppose there are planes leaving for London?' I asked, uncertain what to do and feeling strangely foolish and out of place in this critical situation my friends were in.

'Yes. My wife can drive you to the Airport as soon as we've had breakfast.' He left the room and I went to the bathroom to shave and have a quick shower. While I was dressing I recalled how I was once nearly involved in the war against Israel.

That was the 'Six Day War' in June 1967. At that time I

was in Perth, Western Australia, and when the news came that Egypt, Syria and Jordan were at war with Israel, I listened aghast to what Gamal Nasser had to say to his troops on that occasion:

'Kill the Jews and those that are left alive drive into the sea.'

No one in the UN raised a finger in protest. The Russian president asked President Johnson to agree that neither would become involved in the war. Obviously he thought that Israel would be annihilated in a matter of days. No one expressed sympathy, either actively or verbally, for the little nation.

But when to most of the world's amazement, the Six Day War did not result in the Jews being driven into the sea but instead they smashed all three adversaries and the Israeli armies, led by brilliant officers, marched ever onwards, driving their attackers back into their own countries – suddenly the UN found its voice. Now they decreed Israel must be stopped. The war must end as soon as possible. And Israel was declared the aggressor.

So she was forced to stop fighting and a peace treaty was signed. Only few months later Israel was asked to give up the lands she had won by the blood of her soldiers.

I wondered now, would history repeat itself? When my friend came to say good-bye, I had an idea of my own. I told him that once before I had volunteered to go to Israel. But by the time my passport was in order in Australia and I received the visa to go to Israel, the war was over.

Now I was here and there was a war. Why should I run? I asked him to take me with him to the regimental quarters so that I might offer my services to the military authorities.

Yzchak looked at me in disbelief. 'Are you serious?'

'Dead serious,' I said. 'Let me come with you!'

We drove in silence to the military headquarters where he had to report. I was introduced to the Commander, who, after listening to my unusual offer, gave me a friendly smile but explained that I could not join the military because I was not an Israeli citizen.

But he assured me that he appreciated the offer and would record it in his files. He shook my hand with touching warmth.

At first the war went against Israel. They were unprepared,

having settled instead to offer prayers on Yom Kippur in synagogues all over Israel. But no one in the UN had a disparaging word to say against the aggressors. Israel stood entirely alone. The dedicated officers, however, and the soldiers soon turned the tables on the aggressors themselves and General Ariel Sharon's army crossed the Canal and threatened to destroy the whole third Egyptian Army or take it prisoner. Thus the way to Cairo would be his to take.

That was when UN found its voice. 'No,' they shouted. 'Israel must stop fighting,' and once again an uneasy peace was forced on her.

As far as I was concerned, I felt sad that I could not do anything to help. If the war continued I was told that I could work in some civilian hospitals looking after civilian patients as most of the doctors were already in the army.

I did, however, visit Jerusalem and was able to pray in the Church of the Holy Sepulcre. On my way to Jerusalem, we stopped at the Memorial for the Jewish Martyrs of the Second World War – 'The Hand of the Lord' – it was a horrifying sight to see the photographs of the beautiful Jewish girls who were marched nude to their deaths by the Nazi beast. Or the small children wandering perplexed to their annihilation in the gas chambers. And at Massada I stood mesmerised, conjuring up pictures of the Jewish Martyrs who preferred to perish in freedom rather than survive in slavery.

The war ended and I had to leave for London. Either because of my friends' support or because I offered my services to the military, I was given a free passage to Rome.

I had said I wanted to stop there for a few days' rest and so I flew El Al once again. The atmosphere on the return-journey was muted, people seemed disinclined to chat and laugh.

That was nearly a year ago. I was telling my friends in Perth about my Israeli adventure. When I mentioned acupuncture, Stan Irlington suddenly perked up.

'Can acupuncture help me?' he asked.

'I really don't know,' I said. 'But I have seen many people

suffering from asthma treated at the clinic in Vienna.'

'Would you try with me?' he pleaded. 'You said that if when it doesn't help at least acupuncture doesn't do any harm. Isn't that so?'

'Yes,' I replied. 'The professor in Vienna assured us that acupuncture does not harm the patient in any way. He also said that if three sessions do not show any improvement in the patient's condition, the honest doctor must stop the treatment. It would be dishonest to go on with the treatment in such a case.'

'Would you try it on me?' he begged again. 'Please!'

I could not refuse and Stan became my first acupuncture patient. I studied the book written by Professor Johannes Bischko carefully and followed the instructions to the letter.

Stan was lying on his bed with his chest bare. I selected the points on the Meridians that were the ones for asthma. I left the needles in for about half an hour. I told him that we would repeat the treatment in a week's time. Not before.

The next morning I was awoken by an excited voice over the phone. I did not recognise it at first. 'Who is speaking?' I asked stupidly.

'It's me, Stan – your patient,' came the answer.

'Is anything wrong?' I began to worry.

'No, no, nothing is wrong. I feel so much better. I had a completely trouble-free night. I'm breathing like a young man again!'

'I'm delighted to hear it.' Perhaps it was imagination, I told myself. But it was neither imagination nor auto-suggestion. Stan was really feeling better.

I examined him carefully. I listened to his chest. His breathing was almost normal. All the wheezing had gone.

We repeated the treatment twice more. Stan was free of his asthma. But what would happen if he went in the country to his estate again?

We had to try. I suggested we all go – Stan, Max and I. Accompanied by their two ladies we all drove in Stan's Cadillac. We stayed in the country for the whole week-end. We went round inspecting the fruit-trees, the wheat and barley tracts. Nothing happened. Stan's asthma was gone. He insisted that I gave him three more sessions for good luck.

I complied willingly. I was as excited as the patient himself. Stan did not sell his beloved land and orchards. On the contrary, he now spends most of his time in the country. And he always gets in touch with me to assure me that he is really cured.

The last time I saw Stan it was two years later – this last autumn as a matter of fact. He is as well as ever. No more asthma and no more allergies!

As might have been expected, The news of Stan's cure by acupuncture spread like wildfire. He was a well-known personality and his friends marvelled at the miracle.

Consequently I had to treat ten more patients, all friends or acquaintances of Stan and Max. All of them found some relief with acupuncture but the three land-owners and neighbours of Stan benefited the most from the treatment. They also suffered from asthma and like Stan, other treatment had been useless.

'Why not set up practice as an acupuncturist in Perth?' my friends coaxed.

'Perhaps one day.' I smiled. 'When I'm too old for surgery and my hands begin to tremble when I hold a knife. Maybe then I will dedicate myself to acupuncture.'

II

Operation Called 'Lumpectomy'

Medicine can never be the exact science that some people think it should be. If the doctor knew all the facts and laws about the human body, he could never base his decisions entirely upon those facts alone, as the engineer and the physicist do in their own spheres of work.

The doctor's material is a human being, with all the prejudices, ethical and material, that make up the individual human personality. If the observed data point scientifically to one inescapable conclusion that this or the other is the right course of treatment, then it is quite likely that the patient himself will adduce some particular private reason why that treatment is the very one to which he cannot agree.

The grounds may be religious; they may be simply emotional. So, too, in medicine one must sometimes take a course that the basic science of the situation hardly justifies, merely because there are psychological factors that make it highly desirable. Medicine is, as has often been remarked, the meeting place of art and science; but it is also something more – an adventure in the ways of human souls, an education in humanity in its widest sense.

My thoughts were turned that way by the memory of the case of Jennifer. It was a curious case in which scientific necessity and emotional scruples became hopelessly entangled in a way that seemed impossible to unravel. And it was also one of those cases in which the surgeon's knife cut away not merely bodily tissue but also the weeds of unhappiness that had grown round two lives.

In her teens, Jennifer had been one of the beauties of her

year, and when she came to see me, then in her late twenties, she was still strikingly handsome, though there was an air of shyness about her that seemed quite out of character.

I have come to recognise that particular expression. It arises from a feeling of self-consciousness due to some abnormality. The air of unnaturalness about it is due, I think, not so much to its being something alien grafted onto the person's character, as to its being almost exactly similar to the shyness of adolescence – due also to self-consciousness – and thus being quite out of place in a man or woman of mature years. The suggestion of gaucherie about it has none of the natural simplicity of the normally shy and reticent individual.

Jennifer had married some years before, and the match had proved successful in every way. She and her husband were seen everywhere together, obviously happy in each other's company. A couple of years after the marriage, Jennifer had her first child, and, though her doctor was dubious about the wisdom of her decision, she had insisted on feeding the child herself.

The results were now plain to see. I had recognised them at once as the fountain of her shyness. It was a type of abnormality that always induces acute self-consciousness in women, as I have said often elsewhere: hypertrophy of the breasts which often follows the breast-feeding of the child. The immediate cause, I learnt on looking into Jennifer's case, was a disturbance in the secretions of the endocrine glands, the outcome also of the same cause.

Now her attitude towards me, a stranger, was embarrassing enough in its air of withdrawal and fear that I might be criticizing her. But as, led on by sympathetic handling, she unfolded the whole of her story, I realised that it was a very serious menace to her whole life.

This abnormality was producing a state that was starkly psychopathological, for it resulted in a degree of uneasiness that was coming between her and her husband – who, incidentally, as I was later to find out for myself, was an extremely understanding and tactful man, of whom no one, least of all his wife, need have stood in fear.

By the time she came to consult me, she had already

reached the stage when she could not bear to allow her husband to see her naked, while the mere suggestion of the intimate relations of marriage produced a feeling almost of nausea in her. And these were the starting points of possible tragedy.

At first, her husband treated her with consideration, but as she withdrew further and further from him, he began to wonder if there was not something else behind it than mere embarrassment.

Doubts of her continued love for him rose in his mind; and the more she insisted that it was merely her appearance that worried her, the more he felt that this was a mere excuse and that he must look further afield if he was to find the real cause of her changed attitude.

Suspicion is a plant that flourishes quickly once the seeds have been planted, and in this case it did not belie its reputation.

Vague uneasiness deepened into unhappiness, and unhappiness into open discord. The mutual understanding that had marked the early days of their marriage disappeared, and its place was taken by suspicion and mistrust. Each laid the blame on the other. An accusation denied was taken as proof of guilt. The story is too familiar to students of humanity to need repeating in detail. It ran its appointed course until it reached that point at which a decision must be taken – a decision that must set the scene for the whole of their lives. And here there seemed only one logical outcome – divorce, unless some help could be found.

It is a curious thing that two people may quarrel every time they meet and their day-to-day lives together become impossible, but unconsciously the small hope of reconciliation never seems quite to die, and the decision to end it all is rarely taken without reservation and reluctance.

Those who argue that all divorce should be by agreement are probably the strongest advocates of harder divorce and not easier, as they suppose themselves to be. It was thus with these two. They agreed upon the desirability of separation for the moment and not a final divorce. So they could live their own lives. They made no legal deed of separation. For the moment, their future hung in the air, since neither had the courage to take the final irrevocable step.

Young Jennifer was very unhappy from that moment. In the hope of forgetting her sorrows in arduous work, she took a part-time employment with a real-estate agency. But it made little difference to her. Deep in her heart, she knew that she still loved her husband, and she believed that all this would never have happened if she had not become the victim of this glandular disorder which had so transformed both her body and her mind.

How often it happens that the map of the way out is produced only when the travellers have gone too far! It was an ironic tragedy indeed that not until the final separation had taken place and the affair seemed doomed to end soon did a friend of Jennifer's come to her rescue.

This was the one person to whom she confided all the unpleasant details of her acute inferiority feeling. That friend opened her eyes wide with astonishment. She had always imagined Jennifer to be a sophisticated girl to whom most things were known: and it came as a shock to her to realise that Jennifer knew nothing at all about the possibility of a plastic reconstruction of abnormally large breasts.

A new light of hope dawned upon the tortured young woman. Bright thoughts of restoring all that had been lost filled her mind. She begged her friend to make an appointment to see me and to come with her 'for moral support'. Her friend, naturally, had agreed and so both ladies were sitting in front of me in my consulting room.

The examination was encouraging. It was by no means an out-of-the way operation that would be involved. The whole thing could be done, and I had no doubts of the outcome.

I explained that the intervention was not dangerous and it would restore her breasts' contours.

'May I think it over?' she asked.

'Of course, take all the time you need,' I answered. 'It is not an urgent operation from the medical point of view. But in your state of mental depression, I would suggest you do not wait too long.'

'Thank you, doctor, for your kindness.' She smiled and was gone.

But I was not kept on tenterhooks for long. The reply came from Jennifer herself three days later. 'Could I see you soon? The sooner the better,' she begged on the phone.

I arranged for an appointment for the following day.

The moment Jennifer came into the room I could see that she had come to a decision. Nevertheless she was still in low spirits and painfully shy. And above all she was still afraid of the operation. She was beset with the fear that something might go wrong.

I tried to assure her that nothing would go amiss. She was a healthy woman, and although the operation would take nearly three hours to complete, with modern up-to-date anaesthetics, even longer operations did not constitute a danger.

'Thank you, doctor, for being so understanding and frank with me. When can I have the operation?' she asked calmly, to my surprise and with an eagerness I could never have expected from someone as reticent as her.

'I will make arrangements as soon as possible,' I promised. On that note we parted.

I managed to arrange for the operation for the following Friday – three days after our last consultation. I informed her doctor who agreed to assist me. I was glad because he could then also follow the case after the post-operative recovery.

There is no need here, to go into details about the technique of the operation. I expected no difficulties of any kind to crop up. And the operation proceeded smoothly enough.

Just another successful breast-correction, I thought, as I removed over half of the breast-tissue from the patient's right breast and shaped the new, much neater form.

I smiled at the assistant and we changed places.

'It has taken you just one hour,' he complimented me.

'With your expert assistance,' I returned the compliment and proceeded with the work in hand.

We now began to remove the same amount of breast-tissue from the left breast. As usual, I examined the removed portion and felt some hardness in its centre.

'We had better send the whole piece for histology tests,' I instructed.

The operation was completed and the patient wheeled out of the operating theatre in excellent condition. I did not expect any complications in the critical post-operative stage.

'She should be able to leave the clinic in a few days' time,' I told her doctor.

The following two days went by and the patient looked better and happier every time I visited her. And then disaster struck.

On the third day an urgent message came for me from the laboratory to which the tissue had been sent for examination. I couldn't believe my eyes as I read the dreaded word 'Cancer'.

The hard nodule I had detected in the portion excised from the patient's left breast turned out to be malignant. I spoke to the technician and saw the slides for myself. There was no doubt – it was carcinomatous.

What were we going to do? Both the family doctor and I asked ourselves. We consulted an expert on cancer. His verdict was the same. Radical amputation and removal of the muscles of the left side of the chest. Also the glands from the left armpit had to be excised too.

We called the husband and sadly informed him of the calamity. He too, understood that the only thing to do was to bring the patient back once more into the theatre to remove her breast – Radical Mastectomy.

'Poor Jennifer!' I thought. 'What a pity that she cannot at least enjoy her new breasts for a short while!'

The dreaded moment arrived. We had already wasted three days, and we knew better than most that every hour counted. So all three of us – her doctor, the husband and I entered the room where Jennifer lay happily anticipating the joy of seeing her newly shaped, perfect little breasts.

'Why so gloomy?' were her first words as we came in and approached her bed. We must have unwittingly betrayed our anxiety in our downcast expressions.

I decided to be frank and to the point. Jennifer was an intelligent woman, full of life. Surely even a deforming operation was preferable to the loss of her life!

I explained as tactfully as I could and told her that the disfigurement would be not too noticeable with the well-fitted padded brassiere.

She listened in silence, silent tears streaming down her face. Not one word or sigh escaped her lips. Then suddenly she sat up in her bed and looked us square in the face. Once again I saw a different woman. Not the timid, shy, depressed one I had seen on that first occasion; nor the decisive one who was eager to have the operation. This was an entirely new woman facing us now.

She looked first at me; then her gaze focused on her husband. Then she lowered her eyes and beheld her still bandaged but well-shaped breasts. With both hands she caressed those bandaged breasts gently, lovingly.

'Gentlemen,' she said in a strong, commanding voice. 'All my adult life I have suffered from an inferiority complex caused by my large, unsightly breasts. I was on the point of losing my own husband because of it. And now, at long last I have what my heart desired most. I can tell how beautiful and shapely my breasts are. No, Dr Sava, I'm not going to have the operation. I would rather die with my new breasts than live deformed for the rest of my life!'

It was not merely an argument. It was an indisputable statement of fact she had just declared. She knew, she stressed, of all the dangers. She was well enough aware of the hazards of breasts cancer. But still she would not have the operation. And that was final! When she had done, she reclined on her bed with her eyes closed. Only the pathetic trickle of insistent tears betrayed her torment.

We pleaded with Jennifer. I warned her of all dangers and reminded her of her love for her son and husband. Still she would not be swayed. Her husband pleaded, begged and assured her of his ever-lasting love and the unhappiness her death would bring to him and their child. She remained adamant.

Finally there was nothing for it, but for us to abide by her decision. It was her life. She had to sign the usual paper that she refused the operation against doctors' advice.

There was nothing more to be done. Jennifer stayed at the clinic until I removed the stitches. My heart filled with sorrow and compassion. Her breasts were lovely in every respect. Perhaps she was right. Maybe it was better to live a short but happy life than to go on in torment for the rest of one's life deformed.

We never mentioned the cancer operation again. Nor even the shapely breasts which had prompted her to refuse the mutilating operation.

We parted in silence and shook hands. Her grip was warm and friendly. But no words came forth from her mouth.

'Good-bye, Jennifer,' I said. 'Let me hear from you sometimes.'

She did not reply, but left the room in silence, accompanied by her husband.

That was over seven years ago. Did Jennifer die from cancer of the breast?

No, she did not. She is still alive, happy and their family has been increased by another child, this time a daughter.

It was at a party that I met Jennifer again. This time it was Jennifer who spoke first. She informed me of her baby daughter and told me that she did not breast-feed her.

'I could not bear to spoil my breasts. They are still as beautiful as the day you saw them that last time in the clinic.'

We parted as friends.

Jennifer's refusal to obey the natural laws of the events in the case of cancer had a profound effect on my own way of thinking.

I remembered all the patients I had been forced to deform because radical mastectomy was the only method of saving their lives. Of the many who, like Jennifer, would have preferred to take the chance and risk their own lives, but had not had the courage or the determination.

Could I not follow the path on which Jennifer had inadvertently set me?

I determined not to do any more radical mastectomies. I decided to remove only the lump in the affected breast. I called the procedure 'Lumpectomy' – removal of the tumour – not cutting through it, but removing it surrounded by a small thin layer of healthy breast-tissue.

But to avoid complications of any kind, I supplemented the operation with radiation to the affected area and surrounding tissue and arm-pit, immediately following the removal of the 'lump'.

I have on my list five patients thus operated – the last one three years ago. All of them, including Jennifer, who did not have any X-ray radiation treatment, are alive.

Granted, I have had my misgivings. More often than I cared to I was compelled to listen to admonishments against my folly in the adoption of this method.

'One day you will regret your rash decision,' friends would warn me.

Yet I persist in my opinion that a simple 'lumpectomy' followed by radiation is the better course. It gives the same chances of survival as radical amputation and leaves the patient with her breasts intact.

My final reward came last year at a Conference of Cancer of the Breast held at Stanford University.

Several prominent speakers still held to the notion that only radical mastectomy was the cure for breast cancer. But the radiologist at Stanford and many other surgeons brought out cases where only 'lumpectomy' had been performed, followed by radiation. The results were astonishingly better that any other method available.

They all showed patients surviving more than five and even ten years.

My patients were not included in this list, but I had private satisfaction in the knowledge that I was one of the first surgeons to refuse to amputate and deform his patients.

My final advice is: In patients over the age of menopause, 'lumpectomy' is definitely preferable. In younger patients, if the tumour is still small and the glands are not affected, again 'lumpectomy' is the favoured procedure. Only when the cancer has spread and the arm-pit glands are involved, then a radical mastectomy is advisable to prolong at least the life of the patient for a few years.

III

Drunken Driving and the FBI

I left the party with the ring of good wishes for my speedy return still in my ears. That party at a Downtown restaurant was held to mark the end of my four years' work at a small California hospital. All the hospital's medical staff with their wives and many of their friends had gathered to give me a hearty send-off. My work in California, it seemed, was at an end. The next afternoon I was booked to fly home: to England.

Not that I could ever be really sure where home was. I am an inveterate traveller. I suffer from that disreputable disease which the Germans call 'Wanderlust'. They liken it to a fever or housemaid's knee. In my experience it is more like a common cold or influenza. It always seems to attack me unexpectedly and usually at the most inconvenient times. Too often I have found myself leaving one job to take another thousands of miles away in another country. That had to stop now. England was after all my true home and, as I planned it, the next few years, until my retirement, would be spent there. Perhaps some hospital in England would accept my services. Perhaps some old patients who still remembered me would come back to me.

Such were my thoughts as I shook hands with my American friends – the doctors, their assistants and those nurses who had worked with me in the operating theatre – and drove fast, too fast, along the deserted freeway towards my apartment.

As it happened, it was very fortunate that the nurses were among the wellwishers. Most of them had brought along husbands or boy-friends. Susie, my best surgical nurse, had brought along her fiancé, a prominent criminal lawyer, or attorney as he is called in the States.

Alf Kovalsky was of Polish descent three generations back. Now only his name betrayed his origin. For Alf was a typical American in the best sense: generous, warm-hearted, impetuous, perhaps a little loudmouthed, due more to his vocation, I am sure, than to the land of his birth. He was a very successful Beverly Hills attorney, and that is not a bad thing to be. Especially for the attorney himself.

We took to each other from the moment we shook hands. Perhaps his Slavonic blood was akin to mine, who knows? At the party we sat next to each other for dinner and discussed everything except medicine, which to me was a great relief.

'I'm sure sorry you're leaving this country, Doc,' he said in the flattering way Americans have. 'From what I hear you're one hell of a good surgeon and men like you are surely needed here.'

'That's very nice of you,' I replied. 'But your source of information – the delectable Susie, I suspect – is exaggerating. She's a most capable girl, and we formed a very good surgical team. But the hospital has a lot of good surgeons, so one more or less won't make all that much difference.'

'I doubt it,' he said. 'But even so, I'm still sorry you're leaving after we've just become acquainted. I just feel we could really hit it off.'

I admitted to the same kind of feeling myself and wrote my address on the back of my American visiting card. 'Maybe I'll see you in London some day,' I said.

He grew more animated. 'That's quite possible, George. I've been invited by the English Barrister Association to attend their annual meeting. Now I know you live there, I might well accept.'

'Good.'

'Here's my card, George.' He handed it to me. 'Don't forget, if you ever return before I get to London, look me up.'

'I promise, Alf,' I said. And that was how we parted. Suddenly I was woken from my reveries by police sirens. In my mirror I could see flashing red lights telling me to stop.

I really can't explain why I did what I did next. There was

no earthly reason for it, it was pure impulse. True, I had had a few drinks but I wasn't drunk. Yet, instead of stopping, I found myself accelerating immediately I saw my exit from the freeway. Perhaps I half hoped to lose them as I turned off the freeway into the street where I lived.

I should have known better. The Californian police force is noted for its efficiency. Five years in California should at least have taught me that. But the deed was done. As I slowed down, the police-car passed me and blocked my passage so that I had to slam down hard on the brakes.

Two men, obviously enraged, tore down on me. One had his right hand on the holster at the ready, a sight to gladden the heart.

Before I could get out of the car, two powerful pairs of hands dragged me and held me spread-eagled over the hood of my car, busily frisking me for fire-arms. Then they roughly turned me round. That was when I caught sight of the sergeant.

'Why didn't you stop when we signalled?' he yelled at me.

'I didn't realize you were signalling me,' I said. 'I'm a doctor on my way home from hospital.' Two lies in a row.

'You're a doctor?' The sergeant's tone sounded slightly more respectful this time.

'Yes, at the local hospital.' I pointed to the outline of the hospital building. 'You can see it from here.'

He gave me a brief lecture on how a doctor who treats accident cases at a hospital should know better.

I felt it wisest to agree with him before tentatively enquiring what I had done wrong.

'You were speeding, sir,' the younger of the two grunted. 'We clocked you at over 80 miles an hour.'

I couldn't argue with that. Immersed in my reveries, I must have sped without realising it.

'I'm sorry, officer,' I said, stupidly adding that I had been at a party with other doctors and just didn't realise how fast I was driving.

'A party?' repeated the sergeant. 'Hm. D'you mind if we take a breathalyser-test, sir?'

'Yes, I do mind. I'm not drunk. You can't make me.'

Neither could they. But they told me I had to accompany them to the station.

I objected. 'Surely you can't arrest people for speeding? Just give me my ticket and I'll pay my fine.'

'We're taking you in, sir,' said the sergeant, 'on suspicion of driving under the influence of alcohol.'

Further argument was pointless. I was arrested and the law in California requires an arrested man to be manacled. Instead of being snug in my own bed at home, I found myself handcuffed to a couple of policemen at a nearby police station, attempting to explain my side of the whole, sorry incident.

Mercifully the handcuffs were soon removed and another officer took the statement from the two who had arrested me.

The station officer turned to me:

'You're entitled to a lawyer, sir, on a charge like this.'

God, it suddenly dawned on me, what have I got myself into. Aloud I said:

'But I'm not drunk!'

'You refused the breathalyser-test.'

'OK. Go ahead now, if you like.'

'Oh, we will,' he countered. 'But you'll still have to spend the night here. If I were you I'd call my lawyer.'

I was about to say I didn't have one when I suddenly recalled my new friend of but a few hours back. Alf Kovalsky. His card was in my pocket. I took it out. 'May I?'

'Go right ahead,' said the officer, pointing to the telephone.

I dialled Alf's number, silently praying he was home already. Otherwise what? But my luck had turned. Alf's voice came on the phone almost immediately.

'Alf, this is George – George Sava.'

'Well hello there,' chuckled Alf. 'This sure is a surprise. Didn't expect to hear from you quite this soon.'

'No,' I agreed sadly, and told him I needed his help badly.

'You bet ya – what's wrong?'

I explained that I'd been arrested and was at Encino Police Station.

'Ch – rist!' my friend couldn't help exclaiming. 'What the hell for? You don't quite fit the role of rapist or murderer.' It was a relief to be able to laugh.

'Not quite as bad as that,' I said, 'suspicion of drunken driving.'

'Nasty enough, Doc. Don't say a thing. I'll be with you in about half an hour. And George, remember now, don't say a thing!' Then he hung up.

'My lawyer will be here shortly,' I was able to tell the officer. Meanwhile, I sat between the two policemen waiting patiently for Alf Kovalsky.

In twenty minutes, Alf had arrived. I was very glad to note how cordially he greeted the policemen. They had met before.

'The doctor's a friend of mine,' Alf told them. 'What's the charge, sergeant?'

'Suspicion of drunken driving and speeding, Mr Kovalsky.' And he proceeded to read the statement.

Afterwards, Alf slowly shook his head. 'The doctor refused the breathalyser test? The way he was treated I'd have refused myself.' Alf developed at length his theme of the injustice of the police. 'Frisking a self-respecting citizen as if he were a common criminal.'

Finally: 'My client is quite ready to submit to the breathalyser test.'

The test proved negative. The two-hour delay caused by my refusal must have helped.

Alf Kovalsky had a quiet chat with the sergeant about the second charge of speeding. By law I should have been fined and my licence endorsed.

But the sergeant was an altogether changed man. 'Doctor,' he smiled at me, 'you're sure lucky to have a pal like Mr Kovalsky.' According to him, Kovalsky was not only a great lawyer but a great friend. For his sake and 'because we did treat you a little roughly,' they withdrew the speeding offence.

I longed to say a loud 'Halleluja'. Instead, I contented myself with shaking hands all round. The atmosphere was now so amicable, I half expected them to throw another party for me.

Then I noticed the two sergeants having a private chat and now and again, casting looks in my direction. What next? I wondered.

'Doctor,' said the senior of the two, turning to me at last.

'You're a plastic surgeon?'

I acknowledged it, with a smile.

'And a damned good one,' intervened Alf on my behalf.

The sergeant grinned. 'In that case, doctor, would you do me a favour?'

'With pleasure,' I replied, with genuine relief. What was it, wife with too small a bosom? Girl-friend with too large a nose? I joked aloud. 'Surely you're not in need of plastic surgery?'

'No, not me, but a great buddy of ours is.'

I asked for more information

'It's quite a tale. Poor Frank – Frank Waseley, Chief of the FBI in this area.'

'Not Frank,' said Alf Kovalsky in surprise. 'What's the matter with him? We played golf only a few days back.'

Even I had heard of Frank Waseley. On occasions he had come to the hospital on routine police business.

'He's badly burnt and right now he's at the Naval Hospital.'

I explained to the sergeant that meant I couldn't really help I had no rights to operate at the Naval Hospital. They had their own staff.

'I know, doctor,' he said. But I heard from Frank's wife that they'd done some grafting on him and it was unsuccessful. So his wife told me he's asking for another opinion and would like to be transferred. Even J. Edgar Hoover has been in touch with the hospital.'

'Well, if permission is granted by the hospital authorities, I suppose I could see him as a consultant and give him my opinion.'

'Would you, doctor?'

'Of course.' But I expressed an honest doubt about being able to improve on what first-rate men at the Naval Hospital could do.

'Sure, but with you being European-trained and having travelled the world and all.' I wondered what further mysterious qualifications that conferred on me. He went on, 'Anyway, you'll go and see him if they grant us permission?'

'Of course.'

The sergeant looked at his watch. 'It's past two a.m.

Tomorrow I'll have a word with Frank and contact you after, if I may.'

I nodded. I refrained from telling him that I was on the point of leaving for England. A few days longer wouldn't hurt. Even if I couldn't do any better than the plastic surgeons at the Naval Hospital, I could hardly refuse a consultation. So I reasoned with myself that early morning when at last I dropped into my own blessed bed.

Early on Monday morning the phone-call from the police sergeant came through: 'Good morning, doctor,' he said cheerfully. 'I've had a word with our friend, Mr Waseley. He'd be real obliged if you'd come and see him.'

I asked where we were to meet.

'We'll pick you up in about half an hour. Is that OK with you?'

'Sure, sergeant. I'll be ready.'

Shortly after nine o'clock, a police car drove up. Outside the apartment, a very different sergeant from the night before greeted me with a smile and shook my hand.

The Naval Hospital where Frank Waseley was being treated was situated on almost the other side of California. The journey took well over two hours and we arrived there a little before noon.

A young man met us in the corridor. 'Doctor Sava?'

I nodded.

'I'm John Hawkins, assistant to the Department of Plastic Surgery. Dr Allen, the Chief, asked me to offer his apologies. He happened to be very busy right now. But he left instructions for me to assist you in any way I can.'

'Thank you, Dr Hawkins. Perhaps it would be best if you told me all you know about the case?'

'Wouldn't you like to see the patient first?'

I explained that I prefer first to hear the history of the case and the treatment given so far. 'That,' I said, 'brings me that much closer to the patient when I meet him personally.'

'As you wish, Dr Sava. Here's his chart. Shall I read it?'

'Please.'

It was certainly a bizarre story. Frank Waseley, Chief of the FBI for Southern California had taken his young son on a Sunday picnic in the woods, just over two weeks previously. The boy had been given a new kite and was keen to fly it. So father and son had a fine time, running through meadows and trying to get the kite to soar in the sky. It was then that the accident occurred.

The metal string attached to the kite touched a high-power electric cable. The father was holding the kite at the time and he was the one to get terribly burned. The details of the accident were not clear at this stage, but Frank Waseley was unconscious when some passer-by eventually found him, drawn by the child's cries.

Frank Waseley was taken to the nearby Naval Hospital, apparently lifeless. The doctors managed to revive him by stimulating the heart electrically. Three times the heart started to beat, then stopped again. Finally the doctors managed to bring him fully back to life.

The heart beat was now steady and breathing was normal. But examination revealed multiple third degree burns. The worst were in the palm of the right hand, the one which had obviously held the kite-string.

'It's a miracle,' the young doctor said, as he finished Frank's medical history, 'that the man's alive to-day.'

I agreed with that. Frank Waseley must look, I thought, as if he'd been through hell. I asked what had been done by way of treatment.

'Dr Allen cleased and debrided the dead tissue of the burns and last week we treated his hand by grafting skin on the burnt area.'

'How is he progressing?'

'I'm afraid the skin graft hasn't taken. The whole graft has sloughed off and we're back where we started.'

'Does Dr Allen plan to do more grafting?'

'He had originally planned to. But now the patient insists on another opinion. That's where you come in, Dr Sava.'

I knew of Dr Allen by name. He was a well-known plastic surgeon. I couldn't imagine how I could improve on his work.

But I had agreed to see the patient and could hardly back out now.

Frank Waseley was a man of about forty-five years of age, tall, handsome, with the determined face of a clever policeman who could, if need arose, be ruthless. But my chief impression was one of honesty and sincerity. I felt an instant liking for him.

'It's real nice of you to come, doctor,' he smiled. 'I've heard of the circumstances which brought you here. The sergeant is an old pal of mine and I guess he couldn't resist the opportunity of bringing in a plastic surgeon from Europe.'

I felt obliged to tell Mr Waseley that under Dr Allen he was already in very capable hands.

'Sure, I know Allen is a good man – but I want a second opinion.'

He turned to Dr Hawkins. 'No reflection on your boss, doctor. I've been treated real well here. But Dr Sava is from Europe and I thought he might have some new ideas or techniques.' He was clutching at straws.

I smiled sadly and turned to the young girl at his side. 'Let's see, nurse, shall we?'

The nurse proceeded to take off the bandages very gently.

The sight which met my eyes was far from encouraging. Over half the palm of the patient's right hand was completely gone. I could identify the exposed tendons and joints of the bones. The same dismal picture was presented by the burns of his breast and feet. A large portion of the skin and subcutaneous tissue of the left breast was gone and I could see some of the muscles sloughed off. Both big toes had skin missing on the internal side, right down to the bone-structures. There were other burns of legs and thighs but they were more superficial and did not present such immense difficulties since only skin had been burnt.

It took me over half an hour to examine and re-examine the affected areas, mentally calculating what might be done.

I turned to the young doctor. 'May I have a word with you, doctor?' And to the patient, I said, 'I shan't be a moment.'

Outside I told Dr Hawkins I'd have to speak to his chief or to the Superintendent, if I was to take over the case.

Dr Hawkins said:

'I'm instructed by Dr Allen to tell you that you are most welcome to take over the case. Unfortunately hospital regulations do not permit outside doctors to operate here. So you'd have to take the patient elsewhere.'

I formed the distinct impression that they would be relieved to have the patient off their hands. The failure of the first skin-graft operation must have discouraged them.

I nodded. 'I know the rules. Let me have another word with Mr Waseley.'

After I had explained my position to him, Frank Waseley smiled with genuine delight. 'Then you're taking me on, Dr Sava?'

'I'd like to try. But I've resigned from my hospital just prior to leaving the country so we'll have to find another hospital where I can operate.'

Frank Waseley had already thought of another hospital. A friend of his knew the owner of a small one nearby, who would be delighted to have me work there, 'As a matter of fact,' he said smiling, 'knowing that you'd not be able to treat me here, I took the precaution of asking the owner to come and meet you here. Just in case you agreed to take me on.'

It had all been worked out meticulously.

The sergeant introduced me to the owner of the hospital in the lobby. He said he had heard of me and was most happy to admit Mr Waseley to the hospital in my care.

So, instead of flying to England, I found myself once more a temporary surgeon, this time at Santa Clara Hospital. This was a small but up-to-date institution. I inspected the operating theatre and was glad to note that nothing was lacking in the way of instruments and anaesthetics. The patient was transferred that same evening.

That Frank Waseley needed help was obvious to a blind man. But what kind of help I should give was not yet entirely clear even to me. That night, I lay awake in my bed, reviewing the case over and over again in my mind.

The doctors, having cleansed and debrided the wounds, had performed free skin-grafting on the palm of the right hand. That was standard practice according to the text-books. But the skin-graft had been a failure. Any experienced plastic surgeon knows that a free skin-graft on exposed tendons and bones cannot take because there is insufficient blood-supply with which to nourish the graft. To repeat the procedure would be senseless. Worse, a recipe for disaster.

The alternative, again according to the text-books, was to make a pedicle-skin graft. This necessitates the damaged hand being attached to another part of the body. The skin-flap is stitched to the wound of the hand while remaining attached to the body for blood-supply over a period of several weeks. The skin-graft would most likely take. But the hand would then never be one hundred percent normal again. Frank Waseley was an active, energetic agent of the FBI. Unless his right hand returned to one hundred per cent normality, he would be compelled without a doubt to retire from his present job.

I suddenly decided to gamble on a particular technique. Why had this not occurred to the able American surgeon? The answer is simple. The technique was a very risky one and not acknowledged in the States. And malpractice being what it is in America a surgeon is a fool not to adhere to accepted procedures. No surgeon has a leg to stand on if he is sued for malpractice after applying a technique not officially recognised. You can't blame them for adhering to well-established procedures.

My decision was bold, it had to be. But if I didn't take the risk, I might as well steer clear of the case altogether.

Next morning, I visited Frank Waseley and explained to him in detail what I planned to do. It was a technique, I admitted, which was not recognised in California. If it failed I would be open to fearful criticism.

He understood. 'I'll sign a statement, doctor, saying I agree to the treatment and won't hold you responsible if it's unsuccessful.'

I was very relieved. 'If it fails,' I promised, 'I'll not charge you a dime. If the worse comes to the worst, we can always return to the standard treatment.'

'Cost is no object, doctor,' Frank Waseley said. 'Mr Hoover, my boss, is underwriting any expenses incurred. And,' he added with conviction, 'I've a feeling you're going to succeed.'

The operation was fixed for the following morning.

The technique, known in Europe as the French technique, is also known as 'sliding flaps procedure'. In simple terms, you have to mobilise all the available healthy tissues around the defect and slide them against each other to cover it.

I began with the hand. The healthy portion of the palm was completely detached from tendons and bones, thus producing a flap. I stretched this flap as far as it would go across the wound. Bringing thumb and small finger as near to each other as possible, I managed to suture the flap to the opposite edge of the wound and cover it completely.

The same procedure was repeated on the left breast. This was far easier because the tissues of the breast-wall are more plentiful and more flexible. I brought them together and sutured them to each other. All other superficial burns were dealt with in the same way.

For the big toes I had to revert to the established techniques. There was not enough tissue to moblise and bring together. Therefore I cut out two pieces of full-thickness skin from the abdomen in the shape of the wounds on the toes and sutured them over the defects. The patient was well bandaged and I was left with nothing to do but pray.

The results were far better than I dared to expect. All the wounds healed completely. Two weeks later, the stitches were removed and the patient was ready to leave hospital.

A month of physio-therapy and massage and Frank Waseley was practically normal. Three months later, he was back at work and I was invited to attend a shooting display. His performance was first-rate and he used his right hand as if there had been no accident.

The result for me was a life-long friendship with Frank Waseley and a letter of commendation for my work from J. Edgar Hoover, the Chief of the FBI. It also brought me a new job at Santa Clara Hospital. Temporary, of course. For me, it had to be.

IV

Daphne's Ordeals

Weeks after I had planned to return to England, I was still in a California hospital, putting the finishing touches to the reconstruction of the injuries of a man from the FBI.

In the modest Santa Clara Hospital the case became something of a legend. It did me no harm. Whenever I passed through the corridors of the hospital, nurses and doctors greeted me with the kind of friendship that can only be found in California. In their eyes, I was not some kind of an outsider of distinction. Simply a friend who had been able to help a fellow human being where others had failed. And that warmed my heart.

But now my time was up. Almost a month had passed since I took over the case of Frank Waseley. And today was the day of the final examination. However badly bitten by the wanderbug it is a matter of conscience with me never to move on until my patient's recovery is complete. Now I was free to go.

With the FBI Director's letter of commendation in my pocket and with the good wishes of the patient and his wife singing in my ears, I was once again on the point of departure. As before, my flight was booked for the following day.

Then pandemonium at the hospital. The intercom urgently summoned the doctors on duty that day.

'What's wrong?' I asked a young nurse as she hurried by.

'Terrible automobile accident, doctor,' she replied without stopping.

Well, I said to myself, this is not your concern. I could see, after my month's work there, that the hospital was not short of good doctors and surgeons. If a Californian surgeon can take pride in anything, it is in his efficiency and skill in dealing with road accidents. The countless freeways and highways guarantee that he is never short of material to keep his hand in. My feeling of unconcern did not spring from callousness but from confidence in the doctors around me.

But I was needed, after all. Even as I was shaking the hands of my patient and his wife a second time, I all but collided with the hospital's superintendent. He, being the owner of the hospital as well, had been extremely helpful in giving me every possible facility where Frank Waseley was concerned.

'Oh, thank heavens, Dr Sava.' The man heaved a sigh of relief. 'I was afraid I'd missed you.'

I smiled, a trifle wistfully perhaps. 'As a matter of fact, I was on my way to say my good-byes to you.'

'I hope it's not good-bye, Dr Sava.' There was deep anxiety in his voice.

Somehow I sensed what had triggered off his anxiety. 'I hear you've just admitted some serious casualties,' I said.

'Yes, four of them. But it's the woman among them I'm most worried about.' He didn't want to put the question. 'Dr Sava, would you mind taking a look at her?'

I said I didn't think it was a good idea. Anything I contributed might even interfere with the work of the two fine surgeons already assigned to the case.

'Of course, doctor, they're good men,' he said. 'But they're faced here with an unusually dreadful problem and they need all the help and advice they can get.' It turned out that the two young surgeons themselves had suggested I should be called in on the case. The woman was so badly injured that it went beyond their scope and competence as general surgeons to deal with it. In particular, the patient needed someone experienced in plastic surgery if she was to have the slightest chance of survival.

I patted my breast-pocket with the airline ticket inside and heaved a deep sigh. 'Of course,' I said, 'let's go and see her.' It struck me that I only needed to give whatever advice I could and then leave the patient in their hands.

No sooner had I stepped inside the emergency room and beheld the road-victim in question than I realised that advice of itself would be futile. Equally, at moments like this, all one's personal problems are forgotten.

The woman was so terribly mutilated that even I, hardened as I was to such injuries, gasped in horror. What could I or anyone do to help her?

From the patrolmen who accompanied the ambulance I learnt that it had been a multiple head-on collision on the nearby freeway. Two men had been killed on the spot. Of the four brought to the hospital, three had received less severe injuries and were being dealt with by surgeons.

Daphne Saunders, however, had been left lying there unattended. She was obviously expected to die at any moment because only a nurse was supervising the blood-transfusion she was receiving.

As I came closer I could scarcely discern her difficult breathing. There was a slight gurgling in her throat which presaged imminent death. That the woman was still alive was in itself a marvel, considering the ghastly injuries she had received. As the passenger in the front seat of the car, she had obviously gone right through the windscreen. And her face was such a mass of shattered flesh and bones that not even those closest to her would have recognized her. Even during the war at the time of the heaviest blitz, I had never witnessed anything quite as nerve-racking as this.

A gash right through the left side of her face completely split open the forehead, left eye-region, left cheek and mouth. There were no lips left and a horrible, bloody gap showed where the mouth had been – most likely a soft and pretty one. She was thirty-two years old. Her body was that of a well-proportioned, healthy young woman.

The picture was made more harrowing because her left eye was completely out of its socket as in some crazy horror film.

'My God,' I couldn't help thinking. 'Perhaps it would be more merciful in this case if she died.' But I was a surgeon and my job was to try to heal. I had been asked to help and there was no time to lose. In my stupor and shock, I had already wasted twenty precious minutes in the examination when I should have given immediate orders for the operating theatre.

American efficiency took over. The Superintendent,

confident that I would not desert the case, had seen to it that one of the operating theatres was already prepared. He had also asked the anaesthetist to put the patient under the moment I consented to take the case over. There was nothing for me to do but to change into my scrub-suit.

One of the hospital surgeons who had assisted me on Frank Waseley's case, pleaded with me to let him help.

I told him I needed his help so badly I would have sent for him if he hadn't volunteered. No one could do this job alone.

The patient was already well under and had been draped by the theatre nurses. We both scrubbed hastily, donned gowns and gloves and began the seemingly impossible task of reconstructing what once had probably been an attractive young face.

First, several loose pieces of bone and tissues had to be trimmed and where possible readjusted.

'Shall we complete the enucleation of the eye?' my assistant asked.

'No, leave that for the time being. Let's see first what's pushing it so far out of place.'

Gently, I probed with my finger beneath the eye-ball and felt what appeared to be a loose piece of bone – a piece of broken skull perhaps. Carefully I eased it and took it out. It was not a piece of bone at all, but a piece of glass which had shot through the left temple and lodged itself behind the eye-ball, thus pushing the eye completely out of its socket. After removing the piece of glass, I carefully cleaned a few loose, soft tissues. It appeared that the bony socket of the eye was not deformed although possibly fractured.

Almost of its own accord the eye-ball went back into its socket. I conjectured that the optic nerve and the blood-vessels of the eye were not torn but only stretched. This was why as soon as the foreign body was removed they contracted and brought the eye-ball back into place.

'Well, doctor,' I said to my assistant, 'although it may be damaged beyond repair, we're going to have to leave it as it is.'

After that, we worked for five hours, reconstructing piece by piece and inch by inch, the torn facial structures. Here, too, I departed from the accepted procedure. In cases like this, when the life of the patient is at stake, the usual way of dealing with it is to suture the lacerated parts quickly and allow them to heal. Later, perhaps after a few months, the patient is brought back and reconstruction is attempted.

My own experience has taught me that whenever a case is dealt with in this way, you can never completely reconstruct the organs into their normal shape. Tissues will have shrunk, ugly scars will have formed and the features, in consequence, will be distorted. A life may have been saved, but at what a price. To live in ugly deformity for the rest of one's life.

My method in such cases was to reconstruct completely there and then while the tissues were still soft, while the blood-vessels were still present and the nerves intact. When I outlined my proposal, my assistant was aghast.

'Dr Sava, if this patient doesn't recover, as is more than likely, we'll be sued up to our necks!'

'Sued by whom?' I asked.

'Most likely by the husband who's got away with minor injuries.'

'Look, doctor,' I said a trifle impatiently. 'I didn't ask to do this case. They pleaded with me to take over because I'm supposed to know more about plastic surgery than they do. But perhaps it would be best if I drop out now. The wounds have been debrided and you'll be able to manage without me, I'm sure.' Not being someone who issues simple threats, I was on the point of taking off my gloves.

The young man was even more aghast at my unexpected reaction. He insisted that he hadn't meant to insult me. Only, malpractice in the States made the surgeon's life extremely difficult.

I quietened down. 'I know, doctor,' I said. 'All the same, I'm prepared to take the risk. As far as I'm concerned it has to be my way – or not at all.'

He kept quiet after that. I liked the young surgeon a lot; he was efficient and conscientious. And his reaction was only too typical of Californian doctors. They are terrified, and understandably so, of malpractice suits that run not into thousands but into hundreds of thousands of dollars in damages. This is why they take no risks and stick to the accepted techniques and procedures.

During the five hours of the Marathon, not a single piece of tissue or skin or muscle was excised even when it appeared that there was no blood supply. And finally a face emerged. A face scarred like a geographical map; but a face with broken jaws well-set with lips which looked like lips; with eye-lids and cheeks that looked as they should.

Without the work of the lady anaesthetist we could not have succeeded. I don't know how many pints of blood she gave our patient. In an operation of this kind blood-loss is inevitable. But Daphne Saunders received more good blood than she lost. When at last we took our gloves off she already looked and sounded far better than we could have hoped.

My assistant was elated. In his eyes, this was a miracle that outshone the miracle performed on Frank Waseley. At any rate he wasn't thinking of lawsuits any more as he went to report on the operation to the hospital superintendent.

It had been a pretty satisfying day's work. Not that success was yet complete. A complication I had vaguely feared, did occur. The deep gash on the left cheek went right through the left parotid gland – the main producer of saliva. The saliva secreted by the gland goes through a very delicate duct into the upper end of the mouth between cheek and upper jaw. It is known as the Stenson duct after the man who first described the anatomy of the parotid gland.

Three weeks later, a swelling which had persisted, burst open and the saliva now began to flow freely from a hole in the middle of the cheek. It was obvious that the duct had been severed and the saliva had found a new passage through the skin.

By that time a well-known ophthalmic surgeon from the north of California, a relative of the patient, had visited her several times. After a lengthy consultation with all concerned, I suggested she should be transferred to Stanford University for the specialist to construct a new salivary duct.

To my surprise, I found strong opposition to my suggestion. None of the doctors present, nor the patient and her husband would agree to the transfer. They all insisted that I should undertake the work myself even though I protested that I hadn't sufficient experience in such delicate work.

As Daphne Saunders grasped my hand there were tears in her eyes. 'Look at me, Dr Sava. No one could have done more for me. Please don't send me away now.'

The ophthalmic surgeon added his voice. He said:

'I'm quite sure you're able to handle it.'

Although I was reluctant, I did not protest too long. Deep in my heart, I too wanted to finish the job myself.

Now I needed imagination to guide me. If the duct was damaged, a new one had to be constructed. It's impossible to find the severed ends of the original duct and bring them together. And micro-surgery was not sufficiently advanced at the time.

I had to attempt a new technique. Near the old exit of the duct in the mouth, I bored a channel with a tiny metal rod. It went through the gum of the upper jaw, through the cheek, right into the middle of the parotid gland until the end of the rod came through the artificial canal in the cheek.

A minute synthetic tube was attached to the rod and pulled right through the new channel and into the mouth. Now the hole in the cheek was closed properly and the skin defect sutured, leaving one end of the tube buried in the parotid gland. The operation was completed when the other end of the synthetic tube was anchored on the mucous membrane of the upper jaw with two cat-gut sutures.

All we could do after that was pray the saliva would find its way through this new channel. To my intense relief and satisfaction, it did.

After three weeks, the synthetic tube was expelled automatically through the opening in the mouth once the cat gut sutures which were holding it in place were dissolved. By then the new channel was established. The saliva now flowed normally in the mouth and when the patient left hospital she looked her normal self, or very nearly so. A handsome woman with only slightly visible scars as witness to her horrifying accident.

She was even fortunate with her eye. Mercifully the optic nerve had not been completely severed. For quite a while she did have blurred double-vision which was already improving by the time she left hospital.

A few days later I received a letter of congratulation from the ophthalmic surgeon. He told me that the patient's vision was now almost normal and that he had spoken of me to people at various hospitals where he worked. He promised me that any one of them would be pleased to have me on their staff.

It all added up to a marvellous end to my stay in the USA.

V

R.L. Stevenson's Tomb and Chief Manogha

After a short time as a locum for the Flying Doctor, I returned once more to Perth and readied myself to recommence my travels. I booked a flight on BA for London, via the United States. I intended to stop for a few days in California and revisit my old friends.

A chance meeting and the striking up of a brief friendship with a charming, young couple caused me to change my mind yet again. Their invitation to visit them on their island was irresistible. For 'their island' was that dream island I had read about and mooned about in my youth, thanks to the stories of Robert Louis Stevenson.

Norman Hastings and his wife were living on an estate in Western Samoa. They had their home on the island of Upolu which is a part of Western Samoa.

I met the couple on my lecture to the Women's Club. Norman Hastings was an archeologist and Susan, his wife, a teacher. During the Second World War Norman served with the American Navy and was stationed in the American part of Samoa. These groups of small islands were under American Sovereignty as an unincorporated territory and Norman had served at the naval station on Pago Pago.

Apparently he fell so deeply in love with the Samoa Islands that he vowed to live there some day for good. So, after the Vietnam war he took his young wife there and they decided to settle on the island of Upolu. There they bought a large farm on which they grew cocoa beans and bananas. In addition, large parts of their plantation were covered with coconut trees.

The Hastings had been on an extensive tour of Australia at

about the time of my arrival there. When I met them at the Club, I told them that I had worked in California for several years. I confided also that I was none too pleased with things in Perth and I thought seriously of returning to London.

'I have also,' I said, 'an offer from a hospital in Northern California and I'm going to look at the possibility.'

At a subsequent meeting – a private dinner party as their guest – I showed them the hospital administrator's letter.

'They haven't insisted on a definite date for your arrival,' Norman remarked as he finished reading the letter. Then he handed it to his wife.

'No, they are leaving it to me. But I did not promise that I would take up the offer.'

'That is even better,' Susan Hastings now took up her husband's point. 'Which means you could come and visit us in Samoa for a short while.'

'Yes, exactly.' Norman smiled. 'Please do come. You know our house is on the island of Upolu.'

'Could I really? I mean, could I really visit you?'

'But of course,' enthused Susan Hastings. 'We'll be delighted.'

'You bet,' her husband agreed.

'It's a lovely thought,' I said pensively.

'We'll be leaving in a few days,' said Norman to the point. 'Come as soon as you can. Wire us and we'll pick you up at the airport.'

'I'll do that,' I said as in a dream. 'Yes, I'll do that. In fact, don't be surprised if you see me at your doorstep on your arrival.' We all three laughed at my exaggeration and eagerness and drank a toast to our next meeting in Samoa.

And so this time my route to London via California was to include Samoa. How marvellous, I thought, a few days' complete rest in this tropical island! No more worries, lectures, and above all, no demanding patients. Just lazing under a coconut tree; sipping a long, cool drink and shutting out the world's turmoils; or taking a refreshing dip in the blue lagoon. If this was not bliss, what was?

However, these were not the only reasons which prompted me to accept the Hastings' invitation so impulsively. Their home on Upolu was on the island on which R.L. Stevenson spent his last years on earth. I must admit here and now that I had been envious of Stevenson's travels ever since reading *An Island Voyage* and *Travels with a Donkey*. And that all-time classic *Treasure Island*, still unsurpassed as a fabulous tale of adventure, has haunted my dreams from childhood on.

In spirit I had frequently imagined myself a descendant of the young Scotsman who had captivated my youthful aspirations and who has ever since inspired me with a desire to roam and explore. Perhaps it was my adoration of him and his adventures that has made me the permanent wanderer I have become. I, too, have always wanted to see strange places and meet stranger beings.

I read his *Travels with a Donkey* as a child (and in a foreign language), and I promised myself solemnly that before I died I would investigate some forgotten corner of the globe with the same eagerness and curiosity. Let it be a truly forgotten spot, I told myself, away from any modern civilisation.

In my child's mind I had already selected the spot – the South Sea Islands. I wanted to see Samoa and the hill peak where Robert Louis Stevenson at last found his resting place. And now, after so many decades, that dream was actually to be fulfilled.

How strange that it was a casual acquaintance which was to give me the opportunity. That the Hastings' home should be on the island of Upolu where Stevenson's tomb was! I visualised the words engraved on his tomb-stone. How did it go? I must remember – had I not memorised them ever since I could first read? Ah yes:

Under the wide and starry sky,
Dig the grave and let me lie –
Glad did I live and gladly die,
And I laid me down with a will.

This be the verse you grave for me:
Here he lies where he longed to be,
Home is the sailor, home from sea;
And the hunter home from the hill.

How many decades had passed since I had first read these beautiful verses? Too many. And now I was actually going to see and touch the carving of these unforgettable lines.

'Yes, my friends,' I told my future hosts. 'I'll be with you as soon as ever I can. Perhaps you'll let me stay a few days to see the grave of R.L. Stevenson?'

'Of course, George. We often go there ourselves to meditate. You'll love the hill where he lies – it's quite unique and beautiful.'

'I love it already,' I replied. 'I've loved it all my life.'

And so at last my childhood dream was to be fulfilled. Glorious days of lazing about in warm sunshine were ahead of me. The American friends who had chosen to live in Samoa were as good as their word. Both of them were waiting for me at the airport. After the usual formalities with customs officials, my passport was stamped as a tourist and permission granted for me to explore the islands for three whole months. Of course, I had come for only a few days' rest and planned to fly on to California and then to London.

My friends shook my hand warmly and all three of us scrambled into an ancient station wagon. Norman took the wheel and we headed for their 'home'. That was to be my first surprise in Samoa. Their so-called 'small home' turned out to be a huge, rambling mansion which comprised the main quarters for the plantation owners, consisting of five bedrooms with bathrooms en suite. It reminded me every bit of the lovely houses I had so often seen in California – all modern comforts included. Oh yes, even the swimming pool was evident. Though why a pool when the warm, tropical ocean was only a stone's throw away, I could not for the life of me comprehend.

I was given a good enough reason, however, a little later. The sea was warm and inviting enough, to be sure, but the sharks swimming in it were none too hospitable and frequently very hungry. It appeared they had a particular taste for white people and while the natives could swim in the sea virtually unmolested by sharks, no white person could venture into the ocean unless he swam near the lookers-out who would warn him of any approaching shark in good time. This, at least, was the explanation I was offered by my friend Norman. But I could not help suspecting that a pool was also a sign of prosperity and a social status symbol, just as in the States. Every American, or for that matter, most Europeans, like to keep up with the proverbial Joneses and of course, my friends were no exception. As for myself, not being a very strong swimmer, I was grateful enough to dive into a crystal-clear pool in the mornings rather than having to brave the unfriendly sharks in the sea.

Just as soon as I was comfortably settled in one of the guest-suites, I begged my friends to show me the grave of R.L. Stevenson.

'Of course, George,' smiled Norman. 'I can understand your impatience. Most tourists head straight for Stevenson's grave. But there really are a great many other things to see on the island so that we thought we'd leave the visit to the grave for a little later on.'

'Not too much later,' I begged like an impatient child. 'It has been my childhood dream and I find it really difficult to wait.'

'OK, OK,' laughed my kind friend. 'Will tomorrow be soon enough?'

'Yes,' I smiled, relieved. 'That will be quite soon enough,' I had to admit since I had been there only two days in all.

Susan and Norman were rare friends indeed, who not only did not resent my impatience, but contrived to make themselves as free as possible to enable them to be my guides on our exploration of the island of Upolu.

And then came that unforgettable 'tomorrow'. I found myself walking up the hill where Robert Louis Stevenson lay resting in his grave. His spirit seemed uncannily close as I reverently touched the carving on the stone slab. I did not have to try to read the fading verses because I knew them so well. I simply stood there transfixed, moved as I had rarely been. I found myself reciting the whole verse aloud. As tears of genuine emotion were running unashamedly down my cheeks, I concluded with: *Here he lies where he longed to be; Home is the sailor, home from sea ... and the hunter home from the hill ...* The words had always stirred me particularly because they came so close to my own restless existence. Where would my final home be? I could not help wondering. I too was a hunter and sailor who longed to be home.

It would be almost impossible to describe everything my friends showed me on these magnificent islands. It would require and certainly deserves a separate book. We visited Savaii and Apolina and Manano. Most of these islands are barren and only one third of them are cultivated. The group of islands belonged to Germany before the First World War. After the war, Western Samoa was given to New Zealand as a mandated territory by the League of Nations. It became an independent Sovereign State in January 1962.

Some days after the visit to the grave we flew in a small plane to the American part of Samoa and Norman, being an ex-naval officer, was given permission to visit the famous Naval Base at Port Pago Pago. Even the names of the little islands that comprise American Samoa are extremely romantic – Aunuu, Tatuila, the Manna group. We even visited uninhabited Rose Atoll which is so beautiful and awe-inspiring that I would not in the least be surprised if one day it will become a popular tourist attraction.

Two weeks passed as in a flash and I began to feel dejected at having to leave this earthly paradise. But leave it I had to since I simply could not while away my days here indefinitely. Though I must admit it would have taken very little persuasion indeed. So I began to prepare for my departure and my friends for the farewell party they were holding for me. It appears that throughout my adventurous life farewell parties are frequently responsible for the changes in my plans. This time, however, the farewell party did promise not to take up guise as temptress and remain true to its name.

I bade goodbye to my friends and to the beautiful Islands that I had begun to love so much. 'California and London here I come'!

The party was small compared to most of my other farewell parties. But what this one lacked in numbers it more than made up for in sheer noise and laughter. My American friends were clearly as popular as they deserved to be and all the neighbouring planters came to wish their roving doctor friend bon voyage.

It seems that the island's doctors were also amongst their friends and two young men were introduced to me as the local general practitioners. One was an extrovert, loquacious New Zealander, the other was exactly the opposite. He was a taciturn, handsome native who had graduated in New Zealand. There he had fallen in love with and married a nurse – a lovely young girl – and they had settled on the island of Upolu. It was he who had most sought to be introduced to me.

'I especially asked Norman Hastings to arrange for a meeting with you,' he confessed.

'That's very nice of you,' I smiled in surprise. 'I'm afraid that I'm leaving in two days' time as you've probably heard – but we could have lunch together tomorrow, if you like.'

'Oh I'd like that, Mr Sava.' He beamed, flashing his handsome white teeth. 'Would you do us the honour of having lunch with us? We live on the far side of the island and I'd come and pick you up.'

And that was how yet again my plans of flying to London the next day came to glorious nothing. For the next three weeks, however, I changed my role of idle tourist to the one most familiar and suited to me – that of busy surgeon. Not that I minded the delay. The islands held me in their spell with their incomparable beauty and charm. What did worry me was that now I had become used to indolence, would I take to hard work quite so easily?

Dr Mandi Bunghi was also a surgeon and operated at the local hospital. He explained that he had had some training but not sufficient to perform major surgery. Only such minor ones as appendectomies, hernias and lacerations which he could tackle well enough. Being a native himself he naturally enjoyed all the trust and faith of the other natives. Even the chiefs from the furthest islands would approach him for advice and seek his professional help.

'I'm in a great predicament, Dr Sava,' he confessed, after we had finished lunch. 'I really need your help desperately.'

'How's that?' I asked surprised.

'A friend of mine is here on the island. He is an important Chief. He is in urgent need of an operation and honestly, when I heard of your visit here to Samoa, I thought it must be the answer to my prayers.'

'I don't understand, Dr Bunghi. If your friend requires surgery and you do not feel you can help him surely there must be some other surgeons on the island who could come to his help?'

'Oh yes, there are – especially from the American Base. They either fly over and operate at the local hospital or the patient is flown to them.'

'Well then, why cannot the same procedure be applied to your friend?'

'Because, Dr Sava, he requires a delicate plastic operation and there is not a surgeon on the island who could help him.' He sighed. 'I was even thinking of sending him to New Zealand.'

'Yes, good idea. New Zealand has excellent plastic surgeons.'

'Yes, I agree. But the trouble is the Chief won't hear of it. He won't leave the islands. He wants the surgeon to come to him and that, of course, is quite impossible for obvious financial reasons. So, now that you are here you will help us, won't you?"

As I have already stressed, I was so enamoured with the islands that the slightest excuse for an extension of my stay was more than welcome to me, though I would not have admitted as much to anyone at the time.

'What is wrong with your Chief, doctor?' I now enquired.

'Half his nose has been eaten away with cancer!'

'But I'm not a cancer specialist.'

'I know. But the Chief has been cured of his cancer. It is his ugly deformity only that remains. And naturally it bothers him greatly. He imagines that all his subjects must be making fun of him. His authority has been diminished and he is a very unhappy man. Will you see him, Dr Sava?'

'Yes, of course I will. But whether I can help I'll only be able to say after having examined him.'

'I understand and I'm most grateful. I'll bring the Chief to see you tomorrow.'

And that was how I came to make the acquaintance of the great Chief Manogha. He possessed a heavenly name and lived up to it, for he was the acme of politeness and good-humour. Graciously he called me his son. Tall as a palm-tree, he was lithe and possessed a magnificent physique. His skin was the colour of polished mahogany and apart from his affliction he was a splendid figure of a man. But he seemed vital and energetic enough to battle with his affliction – and a terrible affliction it certainly was, especially for a man constantly in the public eye.

Half of his nose was missing. The Chief had been suffering from skin cancer affecting the right ala of his nose. A none too experienced surgeon had excised the ulcer together with half of the poor man's nose. He had rid him of the skin cancer but had left him with a deformity that was as ugly in appearance as it was grotesque, lending an almost comical caricature to the whole face. I could well feel for the man. It was quite a predicament. And I could understand his anxiety to have his deformity corrected.

I made a thorough examination and satisfied myself that there really was no trace of skin cancer. What had to be done was to reconstruct the missing portion of the nose through plastic surgery and thus give back to this dignified man his natural dignified appearance. I noticed how anxiously his doctor friend awaited my verdict. And as I terminated the examination Dr Bunghi looked at me with such an uneasy expression that I could not help feeling sorry for him.

'Yes,' I said quietly. 'I think I can help the Chief.' Both men's faces lit up perceptibly and I too felt a great sense of relief.

Before I began to explain to the doctor the technique I was proposing to adopt, the Chief took up the conversation. He confessed, with a touching childishness, that he had come to see me because his great and trusted friend – Dr Bunghi – had told him of me. My name and fame, great as it was, he said politely, had not penetrated to his islands. But he promised me that when I had cured him he would speak favourably of me.

I thanked the Chief for his generous words and assured him that I would do my best to help him and make him once again handsome and respectable. This assurance pleased him. He smiled and showed his white teeth and again bowed with a simple, noble dignity.

I told the Chief that I would explain how I was going to help him and his trusted friend, the doctor, would help me in the task. However, the day before the operation the Chief told me that he considered me a friend already and would like to tell me more about himself. Friends must know about each other, he said.

And so I learnt the whole history of his dynasty and the islands from the sixteenth century onwards. The Chief boastingly claimed descent from a Scotsman! The Chief was certainly full of surprises.

'My ancestor,' said he, 'was a certain Scots gentleman. The little we know about him is that he ran away from a big ship where the captain had treated him cruelly. So he cut adrift in a pinnace at night and sailed for the first island he could find. It happened to be the island of my ancestors.

'At that time the island was ruled by a lady, a very capable and charming woman whose spirit is ever with me. She liked the boy and when he grew up she made him headman or Prime Minister, as you say, and he did battle for the islands against all invaders and became a hero, learning our language and our customs and becoming one of us. And finally, after he had shown his prowess, the queen let him fall in love with her favourite daughter and so it happened, when the queen died, the Scotsman and the daughter of the queen ruled the island. I am their distant child,' he concluded.

When the Chief stopped talking, the doctor added that the story is true and the Chief is a very good and great person. He was Chief, spiritual head, judge and hangman of his islands and was very popular.

I agreed with both of them and added that I felt honoured that the Chief had entrusted his life to me. 'I will do my best,' I repeated again. The technique I proposed to adopt in this case, I explained in detail to Dr Bunghi and asked him to arrange for the Chief's recovery at the local hospital.

'You'll assist me, won't you, Dr Bunghi?' I addressed my colleague.

'It will be a pleasure and an honour, Dr Sava,' beamed the young doctor enthusiastically.

The technique I intended to adopt was very simple. I would excise a portion of one of his ear lobes in the shape of the missing ala of the nose. Then, after excising also the scars round the nasal defect thus making them bleed, I would stitch the lobe portion onto the nasal defect. With luck the piece of ear will heal in its new place and the patient will have a normal new nose with only a small scar visible. 'Of course,' I explained to the doctor, 'this technique is simple but sometimes it fails. Should that unfortunately happen, we can revert to the alternative technique or raising a pedicle skin graft from one of the chief's arms, bringing the arm near the patient's face and stitching the skin pedicle onto the nose. That means the patient has to keep his arm lifted up to his face for about four weeks until the skin flap has healed to its new place. Then we will have to sever the skin from the arm, re-shape it, and complete the operation. It is a difficult procedure and requires at least two months for completion.'

'I understand, Dr Sava,' said Dr Bunghi. 'Let's hope the first technique will be successful.'

'Let's hope, indeed,' I had to agree.

I decided to give the Chief a local anaesthetic. I mention this because of his childlike innocence. He simply could not understand how he could be cut into pieces and still not feel any pain. It was a great novelty and he even wanted me to operate on him again and again simply for the joy of the thing.

'How is it you do it?' he asked.

'Syringe ... water ... prick in skin and ... no pain,' I explained carefully, demonstrating with my hands. He asked Dr Bunghi in his own language what a syringe meant, and then argued with him for some time before he understood. The water and the prick in the ear and the nose and 'no pain' he followed in English. It appeared that he understood English, but was too shy to try it out on me. Towards the end of the week, when he was well on the way to recovery, I prevailed on him to talk English to me.

As far as the result of the operation was concerned, we were indeed very lucky. The piece of ear-lobe healed perfectly onto the nose and the chief got a nose as shapely and serviceable as ever before. The Chief was immensely pleased with his appearance. He shook my hand vigorously and, smiling, began by thanking me for what I had done for him and regretting that I would not agree to perform any further operations on him. Then he struck on a bright idea.

'Come ... Manogha ... me Chief Manogha ... big island ... You prick Chief Manogha and cut him up ... No pain ...'

I told him how much I would have enjoyed going to Manogha, where he was Chief, but there were no further operations necessary, and besides I had to fly far away to England where I had my duties to attend to.

Chief Manogha was very mournful and began trying to seduce me.

'Have plenty wives ...' he suggested. I told him that I sympathised with him, but he did not understand my reluctance to accept the offer.

'Give plenty wives you ... coconuts and pigs ... You very happy Manogha Island ... sun ... many sharks to catch ... not much work ... You can prick and cut my people. I let you prick as many as you like. I pay you much ... pay with copra ...'

What was copra, I asked. I knew vaguely, but I wanted a better definition.

'Copra? Copra come from big coconut from big trees on island. Big fruit, ripe ... fall down, cut pieces, dry sun, very, very hot sun ... copra!'

Ave Caesar! I mean Julius. He would have envied this laconic explanation or been annoyed at the similarity of style: *Veni, vidi, vici* – copra!

'No,' I said, 'I would not know what to do with copra.'

'Lots of copra I give you. You sell to Americans on ship, they give you plenty of money.' He beamed again, flashing his white teeth. 'We happy people. We eat, drink, and catch sharks ...'

Then he tried another strategy on me. He told me how he used to go shark-catching in his youth. Apparently in

Manogha this sport was as popular as fox-hunting, although a little more dangerous. 'Big prick for shark ... him die ... no pain,' parodied the Chief of my explanation of local anaesthesia. 'You like catch sharks?'

I confessed that I hadn't tried.

'Ah,' he smiled, 'Manogha – you come there and I teach you catch sharks and other fish too. You must come ... one day!' Then he gave me his card. This read beautifully in a comic-pathetic way: 'Chief Manogha Island, Big House in Centre. Ship call once every three months ...'

I promised faithfully I should one day visit him, and he said how glad he would be to receive me and asked me how many years I would care to live with him. I could not tell him for sure.

'I will come, Chief Manogha. I promise ... one day, but not now. Then you can kill many baby-pigs and fish and we will drink our health in coconut wine.' I promised and at that moment I meant it. With that, we parted.

'I hope you'll really return, Dr Sava,' said my new friend Dr Bunghi, who had been silent during the extravagant temptings of Chief Manogha.

'I would like to return very much, Dr Bunghi,' I said with sincerity.

The Chief returned to Manogha shortly afterwards, complete with his new nose. 'My people, when they see my new nose,' he said, 'they will all want to be cut by you. You come, Dr Sava, you come to Manogha.'

I repeated again that I'd try to return and visit him on his beautiful island. That evening I dined alone with my hosts. The next morning I boarded the plane that was going to take me back to London. Would I be happy there? Who knows.

My ears were ringing with the call of Manogha, where the islanders swam in the lagoons and stayed in the sun and grew brown and laughed as little children.

I saw in my mind's eyes the island with its star-shaped shadows of palm-trees and its lagoons where rainbow-fish that were 'flabby' and moon-fish strolled round the coral reefs.

Perhaps I should have accepted the Chief's invitation and remained on his island, where I would learn to dive into the water and hide there until I spied a lurking shark enjoying itself in the warm water.

Yes, perhaps I should have accepted the Chief's invitation and remained on his island for the rest of my days!

VI

Chinese Herbs and Skin Affliction

'No, I must admit, I did not believe in legends, myths or fables,' my companion, whom I met on my stop for a few days' sight-seeing in Tahiti, assured me emphatically as we sat on the veranda of the Bali Hai Hotel in Moorea, enjoying the cool breeze coming from the lagoon.

'You mean to say that now you have changed your mind about legends?' I smiled at him as I gazed longingly upon the exotic island spreading like a giant pearl in the blue ocean. Yes. I mused to myself, this has been an exotic, romantic journey right from the start.

I was on my way back home to London, after attending medical conference in Sydney, Australia.

Originally I had intended to revisit places I knew in Australia from my previous visits there. I saw again Alice Springs from where I made a car journey right up to Darwin some years previously.

It took a boat trip from Darwin, stopping at every port on the West Australian Coast until we reached Perth. There, I was told that the friends with whom I intended staying were themselves visting the States. Disappointed, I decided to cut short my stay in Perth and instead booked a seat on a Pan American plane bound for Tahiti and San Francisco. I still had a few days remaining from my month's leave of absence from my work in London. So, what better way than to spend those few days in Tahiti and then finish my holiday in San Francisco?

Tahiti, the most romantic place of all Polynesia. I conjured up in my mind's eye pictures of palm trees and thatched huts framing a lagoon at twilight. Exotic dancers and sun-worshippers entertaining you while you sipped your cool Tahitian cocktails. It was the French impressionist painter, Paul Gauguin who first gave the Western World much of its longing for the South Seas.

I well remembered his description of the Tahitian girls: 'In her ear, which was listening to the fragrance, she had a flower.' That's how Gauguin wrote about the Tahitian beauty who first caught his attention. And he must have known what he was talking about, spending as he did, the rest of his life painting the exotic landscapes of Tahiti and making love to exotic creatures.

Knowing all this, I could not resist the temptation of breaking my journey for a few days to visit this earthly paradise. This is true not only of Tahiti but of all Oceania. There is so much beauty and such a variety that the senses become confused.

You watch plants growing literally; touch the swift onrush of evening dark; smell the approach of rain and hear the shrieks of jungle birds as if their notes were written on a musical score.

The lure and legends are native to the South Pacific, to the high islands created from volcanoes and the low atolls born of the skeletons of numberless coral polyps. Who could blame Paul Gauguin for forsaking his native France and spending the rest of his life there ? Certainly I did not blame anybody who had the opportunity and the means of living in Tahiti. Nor would I have minded had I the free choice of where to spend my remaining years. But the average man has obligations – the average man is no Paul Gauguin.

No, I only spent a few days there, but those few days will remain unforgettable for a lot of different reasons.

Oh yes, I did meet Tahitian girls and listened to their songs and watched their dances.

The plane landed gracefully like a giant bird and I came ashore on Tahiti, at Papeete, a metropolis in oceanic, Polynesian terms.

I am told that some people don't like Papeete. I fell in love with it from the moment I set foot on its shore.

'Is that your first visit to Tahiti?' A voice startled me from my day-dreaming. Turning towards the intruder of my dreams, I beheld a smiling, middle-aged man in tropical outfit.

His bronzed face spoke of long living under the hot Tahitian sun, but he was not a native of the islands. He was unmistakably a European like myself, who had found ways and means to stay here instead of returning to from wherever he came.

'Yes, it is my first visit to Papeete and Tahiti for that matter,' I answered his question. 'I just flew in from Australia and was admiring this wonderful place.'

'Are you leaving again with the plane?'

'No, I'm staying for a few days before flying to San Francisco.' Are all Tahitian dwellers as curious as this one, I wondered. But I did not feel annoyed or upset at the uninvited intrusion. Perhaps it was all to the good. He might be able to suggest a good hotel to me.

'A wise decision. No man should be allowed to proceed on his travels without seeing our islands,' the man said with conviction. 'Allow me to introduce myself: I'm Dr Georges Moreaux.' He extended his hand which I shook with delight, unable to suppress my grinning.

'A doctor? Of medicine?'

'Yes. Strange, isn't it?'

'Not at all,' I went on smiling. 'Permit me, in my turn, to introduce myself. I'm George Sava, a doctor of medicine!' We both roared with laughter at this quite unusual coincidence, or was it? In this place anything can happen, I told myself.

Dr Georges Moreaux, late of the University of Grenoble, appointed himself as my guide. I welcomed the appointment with pleasure. On his suggestion, I booked not at Papeete's Royal Tahitian Hotel, but at the exotic Bali Hai in Moorea.

'You see, *mon confrère*,' he informed me, 'many people think Papeete is all of Tahiti. They are wrong. It isn't. I'll show you.'

My guide was as good as his word. Taking hold of my small suitcase, he guided me to his ancient Citroën, parked a few yards away.

We drove around the island and I enjoyed the beautiful spots which adorned the whole of the island. We visited the Paul Gauguin Museum where I could admire a genuine painting of the master. Then, as midday was approaching, Dr Moreaux treated me to an excellent lunch, accompanied by local wine at the 'Te Anuanua' – the perfect place to sample local food and atmosphere in its natural setting with no frills.

' "Te Anuanua" means rainbow in Tahitian jargon,' I was informed. 'And now,' my newly-found friend went on, finishing the last drop of wine in his glass, 'we will take a boat and sail to Moorea. I'm a permanent guest of Bali Hai, where you will be staying.'

It was an excellent choice. Moorea proved really to be a retreat from the bustle of Tahiti and the Bali Hai was more than one could possibly wish for. Both tempo and pressure were at a low key and most of the guests were old hands in these waters.

As a rule, I am not a regular church-goer, but the Sunday Mass at the Catholic Church at the entrance of Papetoai Bay, proved to be one that cannot easily be forgotten. Voices boomed, bare feet slapped the floor, and I never heard hymns in rock and roll before.

Was it any wonder that I felt sad leaving this enchanting place?

But, duty calls and it was my last evening with my friend, Georges Moreaux, MD, who was telling me why he believed in legends and miracles. He told me that some six years before we met, he came to the islands to die.

'Yes,' he emphasised, 'I developed chronic nephritis in both kidneys and my colleagues told me that at the most I had six months to a year left.' He smiled happily. 'That, my friend, was six years ago, and as you can see, I am still alive.'

'What has that to do with believing in legends?' I asked sceptically. 'Obviously the diagnosis was wrong. You would be alive even if you had stayed right where you were – Grenoble University.'

He disagreed with me. No, what had happened was this: He had read or heard about the legend of the oldest man on earth. A man called Li Chung Yun, who was born in 1677, living on some exotic island had reached his 256th birthday, looking no older than sixty or seventy years of age. He had outlived twenty-three wives, and was living with his 24th at the time. His regular diet was drinking a tea made of different herbs and tropical fruits three times daily. He did that for two hundred years, and another herb mixture he drank tended to keep him vigorous and alert both in mind and body.

'Surely, you don't believe that?' I laughed.

'Perhaps not quite. The legend must have exaggerated about his real age, but not about the Chinese herb brews.' He nodded his head. 'I came here expecting to die. Then I heard about the legend, bought bags of herbs and dry leaves and here I am – six years and still alive and kicking.'

I looked at him and realised that he really believed in the legend and in the amazing healing teas that were his staple diet.

'Perhaps I ought to try the tea on myself or prescribe it on some of my incurable patients!'

I meant it as a joke, not knowing that fate had already decreed that I would be the man to advise drinking herbal tea to a patient of mine. At the time I drank my last exotic cocktail and said good-bye to my Tahitian doctor friend, the only thought I had was not to miss the plane that was leaving early the following morning.

'*Au revoir, mon ami,*' I bade him farewell, shaking his hand vigorously and genuinely sad at leaving such a good friend.

'*Au revoir, George,*' my friend answered. 'Come again, any time. I'll be waiting for you.'

We parted and he saw me right to the plane. I waved once again and boarded the plane that was going to take me to my next stop – San Francisco. Sad at leaving this earthly paradise, I sat quietly in my seat, fastened my belt and abstained from looking through the window as I had done on my arrival.

The flight to San Francisco was uneventful. I stayed with friends for a few days and then I left for London. It was high time, as I had already overstayed my holidays. No more exotic islands, native dancers, sailing in moonlight and listening to the shrieks of jungle birds. I will return, I promised myself, if only to meet my friend once more and see how much good the herbal teas were doing him.

Next to me sat a young girl, obviously not an American. As I looked at her face, memories of my recent short stay in Tahiti came in a rush.

There was no mistaking the fact that she was a native Tahitian and I could picture her in native dress with a flower in her ear, listening to the fragrance. She might have worn one, no doubt. But now, sitting next to me she was elegantly dressed in modern European clothes, most likely purchased in Paris.

I asked her whether she would like to take my place at the window, but she refused. She too, like myself, did not wish to see the lovely island she was leaving behind. She was beautiful and very young. Judging from her face she could not have been older than twenty-two years or even less. One thing struck me as odd, however, her eyes, large and round and the colour of the ocean round the island of Tahiti, were overshadowed with sadness reflecting profound grief. What could a young and beautiful girl like this one have lost that was worth grieving for, I asked myself.

Ailing she was not, or at least I could not detect any signs of illness. Perhaps loss of some loved-one; perhaps an unhappy affair, perhaps ... but wasn't I becoming impertinent in trying to fathom other people's troubles? Everybody carries in his heart deep emotions of sadness, joy or pain. And everybody is entitled to his privacy.

This self-imposed privacy both on her and my part did not last for long. As is customary, travellers cannot remain silent or withdrawn for long. The very physical proximity makes one wish to communicate, to share one's impressions and even troubles. So it happened with us.

It was she who broke the silence first. She asked me how I had liked Tahiti and how long I had stayed there.

I told her all about my experiences and the unusual friendship with Dr Georges Moreaux and of Moorea and Bali Hai. And, of course, I told her that I was a surgeon and recounted the tale of the legend of the oldest man on earth who drank nothing but herbal teas for two hundred years.

She did not laugh when I said I did not believe in legends, neither did she smile when I said I might one day try drinking herbal tea, but at that moment I did not visualise myself living two hundred years.

I did not ask her why she was leaving Tahiti and how long she had been in San Francisco. She volunteered the information by herself.

I have found on many occasions people will unburden themselves the moment they know their listener is a doctor. This Tahitian beauty was no exception. Quietly she told me that she had been in California for over a year and had visited doctors and specialists both in Los Angeles and San Francisco. Now she was going to London, hoping that somebody there might be able to help her.

I did not ask what was ailing her. If she wished she would tell me soon enough and I would not embarrass her by asking the nature of her illness outright. It might be a secret she did not wish to share with any stranger.

As the journey progressed, she went on talking about her job in Tahiti. She had been working as a dance instructor and dress designer. Dancing she had learnt in Papeete as a child. Then her parents had sent her to Paris to learn dress designing. She had loved her work, but she had loved her island and the people and the ocean more and she would always long to return there again. It was now nearly two years that she had been away from her home.

'What surgery do you specialise in?' she asked suddenly, fixing her beautiful, sad eyes on me.

I told her that my work mostly was plastic and cosmetic surgery. 'Removing scars and blemishes from people's faces and bodies, you know,' I answered, trying to be as casual as possible.

'What about skin diseases,' she wanted to know. 'Have you helped patients with skin diseases?'

'Well, I've had patients suffering from skin trouble, but as a rule, they are looked after by dermatologists.'

There was a silence for a long moment, then, looking downwards, as if ashamed of what she was going to say, she quietly told me that she had been suffering from severe dermatitis for the last four years. Noticing that I was discreetly scanning her face and arms, she smiled and went on. 'My face and arms are all right. It is my body, the lower part, and my thighs which are affected.'

Poor girl, I thought, how much she must have suffered. In her islands people bathe practically in the nude; they dance almost naked and to have festering sores on just those parts of the body which are most exposed in these erotic isles must be an absolute disgrace to the afflicted. No wonder she was grieving so deeply and her eyes reflected the pain with which her heart must have been overflowing.

I heard of her quest for help, of the remedies she had tried to alleviate her disease. She had consulted several dermatologists in Los Angeles and San Francisco. She had twice been in hospital and had been forced to swallow pills and then lie under strong lamps with ultraviolet rays which almost burnt her entire body.

When I asked her if that had helped, she said that the doctors had to stop the treatment because of her severe nausea, vomiting and high temperature. She was told that she was allergic to such treatment and must not try it again.

After two years of search for a cure, she had learnt of necessity to live with her affliction. But she would try once more, for the last time, in London. If that failed too, she intended to enrol at the University in Paris and study for a degree in anthropology. It was fortunate that her parents were well off and she would be provided for after their deaths. She, however, wanted to be independent and as an anthropologist she would be working with people to whom, hopefully, a woman's beauty was less important than the quality of her brain.

I discovered all this by the time we reached London. I volunteered to help find her accommodation and suggested a hotel in Kensington.

She thanked me profusely, said how much she had enjoyed our conversation and even apologised for burdening me with her personal problems.

Suddenly an idea flashed through my brain – veritably a lightning flash. Perhaps it was the influence of my Tahitian doctor friend, or perhaps thanks to my having read papers on exotic cures with acupuncture, herbal teas, having listened to arguments about the validity of cures achieved by nature healers, acupuncturists or herbalists in diseases where orthodox medicine had failed.

I had never, in all honesty, thought seriously about those pros and cons voiced by zealots or detractors. One thing I knew, however. All these fringe medical sciences helped most when the patients believed in them. That was why acupuncture and herbal lotions were more effective in oriental patients and less effective or useless with patients of Caucasian origin and background. In every disease the remedy is more effective when the patient has confidence in his or her doctor.

I have found that holds good even in surgery. How much more confidence then is needed in cases when an unorthodox remedy is tried out. Auto-suggestion plays an important, if not the most important, part in treatment such as acupuncture, herbal teas and, of all things, powders made of reindeer or elk antlers.

The following morning I telephoned my Tahitian acquaintance, who was staying at the hotel I had suggested.

'Maya,' I said, 'I would like to see you, if I may. I have something to tell you.'

'It's nice of you to remember me. Of course, you may. Please come as soon as you can.' The voice sounded genuinely pleased. 'How about joining me for lunch here at the hotel?'

I agreed readily.

After a modest lunch, I suggested we have our coffee in the lounge, away from curious people, where we could talk undisturbed. I told her of my sudden idea of trying something unusual in the quest for a cure for her skin disease. I went on explaining what I had seen of acupuncture being used for treatment of diseases where orthodox medicine had failed. I explained about an article I had read somewhere in a magazine of a Chinese nature healer describing his cures for all kinds of diseases, giving his patients concoctions to drink of reindeer's antlers sliced thin and boiled in water. He claimed to have cured rheumatism, gastric disorders, sciatica and muscular spasms. Even asthma and pneumonia had been cured in patients where other remedies had failed.

On the other hand, skin eruptions, boils and many other afflictions of the skin had greatly benefited from the use of pastes and ointments containing antlers' powders.

Maya seemed genuinely interested in what I was telling her. When she asked whether people suffering from chronic dermatitis had been cured I had to confess that no mention had been made in the article or in other Chinese or Indian scriptures. I also told her that western orthodox medical practitioners did not believe in any of these cures. They claimed that the so-called cures were mostly in the nature of psychosomatic disorders, meaning that the main advantage was only psychological and that there was nothing in these concoctions and 'cures' to justify any claims of real medical properties in them.

I explained that these cures with antlers and herbs had been known to ancient Chinese and Tibetan medical men for thousands of years. There exist Indian and Chinese books describing along with antlers, scores of other folk medicines, traceable to the sciences of ancient Egypt, Babylon and Persia.

For the most part, these were herbs collected at the time when they contained the greatest amount of active medical ingredients – flowers and leaves gathered near bloom time; fruits and seeds at the time of their ripening; roots and plant tubers when in the state of inactivity. The ancient Chinese practitioners said that antlers, when harvested in spring – the period of the animals' mating season, were the best and had better healing properties.

The curious thing, I concluded my oration, is that in present day Russia, particularly in its far Eastern provinces, large deer farms exist so that enough supply of antlers is available and treatment with antlers' decoctions and pastes is allowed.

As with acupuncture, the Orient is full of stories of miraculous cures with sliced or powdered antlers. In Hong Kong, where the top portion of the antler sells for over 500 dollars a pound, anybody can go into the shops of nature healers and order a cup of antlers' tea or buy paste with scraped antlers' powder.

'Do you think I should try this treatment on myself?' Maya asked after remaining silent for a few seconds. 'Do you think it might help me?' She sounded perplexed, almost a little ashamed.

'I think you should try it, Maya,' I answered, looking steadily at her. 'I don't know whether it will help you, but you say you tried every remedy and treatment known to medicine with no help whatever. Well then, what are you to lose? One thing I must impress on you, however. You must believe in this treatment with all your heart. You must by no means feel bashful or ashamed at trying an unorthodox method. You must bear in mind that the evidence for its potency depends on you. On the other hand, I can assure you that in the worst case, if there is no marked improvement, at least it will not have done you the slightest bit of harm. And that is more than we can say about many treatments and drugs prescribed by orthodox medicine.'

'Yes, Dr Sava, I understand all that,' she said in a humble voice. Then suddenly, grasping both my hands in hers, she looked at me. 'Thank you, thank you with all my heart!' Her eyes dimmed with tears which began rolling down her cheeks. She did not try to hide them, because they were tears of happiness and not pain. Like a child, she flung her arms round my neck and clinging motionless, she began weeping in the silent heartbreaking way of the Orient.

I let her weep and unload all the pain in her heart. I remained silent because I felt that no words or gestures would be appropriate at that moment.

Yes, Maya, the Tahitian girl with the flower in her ear, which was listening to its fragrance, was cured of her skin affliction. For three whole months she drank tea made of thin slices of reindeer antlers whenever she felt thirsty and covered her skin sores with a paste made of honey, dry seeds and leaves of Bishop's weed and antlers' powder every night before going to sleep. And her whole-hearted belief in her cure – her absolute faith in this remedy of her forefathers – never wavered for one instant!

By the end of the third month, practically all of her skin

sores and boils cleared but she announced solemnly that she would go on drinking the tea for the rest of her life.

No, Maya this delicate Polynesian flower, did not go to Paris to study anthropology. She returned instead to her beloved Moorea and to her lagoons.

In my mind's eye, I can picture her swimming naked in warm, moon-lit waters or listening to the plants growing. Her happy song would be carried with the swift onrush of the evening dark and join the chorus of the shrieking jungle birds whose own singing notes were written on the musical score of the South Sea winds.

'No, I must admit, I did not believe in legends, myths and fables,' my Tahitian friend's words came back to me.

'Do you believe in legends, now, and miraculous cures?' I felt sure he would ask me next time we met.

I don't know what my answer will be. Maya's chronic dermatitis was cured. That was a fact. Where all modern methods of orthodox medicine failed, an old Chinese remedy succeeded. That was a fact too.

Perhaps it was her fervent, unswerving belief in her Oriental folklore, and her determined will to be cured that were the real remedy. I will never be able to unravel all the factors that went into her cure. Perhaps it is better that way.

VII

Of Guilt Possessed

The sound of broken glass reverberated throughout the whole house and sent a shiver down Anne's body. The attractive middle-aged woman was just putting on her jumper and slacks following her routine morning bath when the noise of the crash came to her ears. It came from the drawing room and filled her heart with knowledge of impending disaster.

Anne lived in a London suburb that prided itself on being one of the few left that could be called genteel and old-fashioned.

Most of the inhabitants were either retired army men or professional people who found the quietness and tranquillity of the district preferable to the hub-bub of the city and the cosmopolitan atmosphere of Kensington and Chelsea. One could still walk in the evenings alone without fear of being mugged or encountering undesirable foreigners whose only assets were their inflated bank accounts.

Anne lived in a small but very neat house with her only son – a little boy of seven. After her husband had deserted the family with his young attractive secretary, she had devoted her whole existence to the boy and her only joy was in the possession of the priceless art pieces she had acquired during her more prosperous days.

Place of pride and honour was of course her drawing room. It was not a big one and combined both sitting room and dining area. As a matter of fact, it was she who after buying the house, had insisted that the separate sitting room and dining room be combined into one larger and more airy.

The French windows on the farther side opened into the

small garden and gave access directly to the hot-house where old Mike, the gardener, grew enough roses and carnations for Anne's drawing-room vases.

She would have preferred a larger house, and the room was not big enough when she occasionally entertained guests, but what it lacked in size it made up in tasteful luxury. The walls were covered with Chinese silk and sported three or four original paintings. The mantelpiece over the Adam fireplace was decorated with small but exquisite pieces of art. Pride of place and honour was given to the Chinese vase that stood in the middle of the mantelpiece. It had been an object of joy to Anne ever since the day she had bought it at an auction at one of the manor houses that were forced to sell their furniture and contents. The vase was about fifteen inches high and on its dark-blue contour hand-painted dragons all in genuine gold were artistically displayed. She was told by an antique dealer friend that it was a genuine antique vase worth many times the price she had paid for it.

Besides herself and her son, the only other inhabitants of the house were a little bright yellow canary that always chirped whenever its mistress came into the room to feed it, and Blacky, the cat, which from jealousy or instinct did not particularly cherish the idea of cohabitation with the bird. Those two most certainly were life-long enemies and it was not difficult to see in the cat's eyes the murderous desire and the watering mouth anticipating a succulent meal.

No, those two creatures could not be left alone in the room. When the canary was left free for its cage to be cleaned and replenished with fresh food and water, Blacky was kept shut in the boy's room. Only after the bird was safely in its cage was the cat allowed to come into the drawing room and purr for a while on its mistress's lap.

The moment, however, the cat entered the canary's chirping would stop abruptly. No, there was no love lost between these two creatures. Although mother and son loved both the canary and the cat, there was a slight difference in their affection for them. Anne, if anything, preferred the cat, while Simon, her little boy, showered all his love and attention on the canary.

That, naturally, made even more pronounced the enmity and rivalry between cat and canary. Looking at them and observing their behaviour, I could not help comparing them to the famous characters of Disney's movie.

I will always remember the day and the date of the disaster that befell both mother and son, and this for more than one reason. But let me relate the events as they succeeded each other.

The crash and noise of broken china brought Anne rushing downstairs, and what she saw in the room made her heart miss a few beats. On the floor in front of the Adam fireplace, lay scattered in profusion practically all the ornaments that had graced the mantelpiece.

With horrified eyes she beheld her precious Chinese vase broken to smithereens. In front of the mantelpiece stood little Simon, her son, also horrified at the sight of destruction.

'You little monster,' the mother shouted at the boy, her eyes full of fury. 'See what you have done, you, you ... I could kill you for that, I ...' her hand lifted above her head, ready to strike as she approached the frightened boy.

'No, mummy, no. I didn't do it. I did not break ...'

His large, beautiful hazel eyes dimmed with tears and his right arm raised to soften the impending blow. It was too late. The infuriated mother's hand came down with force, slapping the boy square on his face. He tilted backwards, tripping over the chair that stood right behind him. Falling over, he crashed heavily on his right, uttering a cry of agony and pain.

'Oh, mummy, I didn't break the vase, honestly I didn't ...' were the last words the boy uttered, and then lay still on the floor.

At that precise moment, old Mike, who heard, or more likely saw from the garden what was happening, rushed through the French window into the room. But he, too, was too late to save the boy from punishment.

'No, ma'am, no. The boy did not break the vase. He was with me in the garden and we saw the cat jump towards the bird. The cage swayed and it must have knocked down the vase.'

'What was he doing here, then?' Still not believing in her

boy's innocence she suspected that the gardener wanted to protect him. She knew that a real friendship existed between these two.

'It's God's truth, it is, m'am, so help me. The boy rushed in through the window trying to shush off the cat. We realised what would happen when we saw the cat jumping all over the cage stand. It should not have been left so near the mantelpiece.' Old Mike shook his head gravely.

'Oh, I'm sorry, Simon, please forgive me. I'll make it up to you, I really will.' Now genuinely repentant for her actions, Anne approached the boy, who was still on the floor whimpering quietly.

'Come, darling, let me look at you. Did I hurt you very much?' She tried to lift the boy but as she got hold of his arms the boy shrieked in agony at the touch of his right arm.

'Don't, mummy, don't. It hurts terribly.' He tried to get up by himself, using only his left arm. And as he finally stood up he tried in vain to raise his right arm. 'Oh, mummy, I can't move it, I can't move my arm.' Tears were continuously streaming down his pale cheeks and his voice was interrupted by his crying which he was unable to control.

Now truly alarmed and repentant for what she had done to her little boy, Anne telephoned me at my house and begged me to come at once.

'Simon,' she said, 'my little boy, you remember, is badly hurt, I think. Please come, Mr Sava, hurry I beg of you.'

There was the unmistakable anxiety and fear I have so often seen in mothers about their children. Mother love never errs when the health of her child is concerned. I did not ask any explanation as to what was wrong with her little boy. I knew only that it must be very urgent and serious, otherwise she would have called her family physician, instead of me.

I knew Anne and her ex-husband quite well, both socially and professionally. Both of them have been at one time or another, patients of mine. Some years ago I repaired a small hernia of her husband's because it interfered with his horse-riding. Anne had consulted me on several occasions and I did a minor operation on her by removing rather a nasty-looking brown birth mole from her back, which both I and her family doctor considered might become malignant in time.

Little Simon was also not a stranger to me. At the age of three he had fallen from the pony his father had given him for his third birthday. Wishing to show his father that he wasn't afraid, he tried to jump a rather high fence and landed in the bush terribly bruised and with a rather ugly cut on his forehead. I repaired that cut by putting in a few stitches and closing the wound. The little fellow, still wishing to show both to his father and to me that he was brave, agreed to have the injured part stitched only under local anaesthesia instead of the general one I would have usually administered in children of that age. From then on we became friends and I was often invited to the house.

Needless to say, I was surprised on hearing of their separation and not a little saddened. For their marriage seemed to be working well and if I had been asked to name a happy couple amongst my acquaintances I would not have hesitated to choose them. But human nature is fickle and often unpredictable.

During the last three years, following their divorce, I had little opportunity of seeing either of them. Her former husband and his new bride moved away from London and Anne and little Simon, being of strong body and healthy mind, did not need my services as a surgeon. Once or twice I visted them for a quick cocktail, but she did not entertain as often as she had been accustomed to.

In less than an hour I was at their home examining little Simon. During the examination I was told what had happened and I had to calm the mother more than the boy. He, as on the previous occasion when I stitched his forehead, was brave as ever.

I examined him carefully and reached the conclusion that he had broken his right upper arm by falling over the chair onto the hard floor.

'Oh, God, what have I done. My poor child. Can you ever forgive your foolish mother?' Anne was crying behind me when she heard my diagnosis.

'Don't worry, mummy. It's nothing serious. Is it, Dr Sava?'

'No, Simon, it is not serious,' I smiled at him. 'I have to take you to the hospital, take a picture of your arm and then set it well and put it in plaster. You won't mind me doing that, will you?'

'No, I won't mind. And I will be excused from playing football, won't I?'

'Yes, Simon. But not only from football. No swimming either.' I knew from his mother that he was an excellent and very keen swimmer.

'Can't I swim with the plaster? I can swim with one arm and hold my broken one outside the water.'

'No, Simon, you cannot.' I smiled again and patted his curly head. 'And now, let's drive to the hospital. We'll have to X-ray your arm, see exactly where it is broken and how bad it is. And then I will put your arm in plaster.'

'Shall I call an ambulance?' Anne asked.

'It won't be necessary, we'll drive in my car. The hospital is not too far away from here.'

Gently, I put Simon's injured arm in a sling and fastened it over his head. Then we three – his mother insisted on coming along – drove slowly to the hospital. I had telephoned the X-ray department of the hospital that I was bringing a boy with a suspected fracture of his right upper arm.

We shortly reached our destination and a few minutes later Simon had his arm X-rayed. As suspected, the X-rays confirmed my diagnosis, but it proved to be not as bad as I had feared. His right upper arm was broken at about a third-level from the elbow and seemed not too badly displaced. I asked the boy whether he would like me to put him to sleep while I set his arm properly.

'No, sir. I don't like general anaesthesia, and I like to watch how you do the plaster.'

'It will hurt, Simon. I have to manipulate the arm, that is, I have to move it one way and the other and pull at it. It will hurt you, my boy.' It was no use. He was determined to show how brave he was. Even his mother's entreaties could not make him agree to a general anaesthesia. I knew, however, that setting a fractured limb can be very painful and I did not wish to subject the little boy to it. I decided on a compromise.

'Simon,' I spoke to him again. 'Do you remember when I

stitched the cut on your forehead? You were a very little boy, then, but you might remember how I did it.'

'I remember, doctor. You gave me some kind of injection and stitched it with a needle.'

'Do you really remember all that? You were only three years old, that's way, way back.'

'Yes, but I do remember, I do really.'

'All right, Simon. I believe you. Won't you let me do the same now with your arm?' He nodded his head in agreement.

The rest was easy. After injecting the skin and muscles round the line of the fractured bone, I waited for a few minutes and then set the fracture. The boy winced once or twice but said it did not hurt him. Not too much.

One more control X-ray to confirm that the fracture was set well and then a full-length plaster-of-Paris bandage was wrapped round his arm which was bent at the elbow. A neck-sling completed the treatment and we drove back to their house.

During the whole of the procedure, his mother insisted on being present, to which I agreed. It would be a comfort for the boy to have his mother near him, I thought to myself.

On their insistence, I stayed for dinner that day and when I left them round about ten in the evening, Simon was already snugly asleep in his bed. I told his mother that the plaster would have to be changed in two weeks' time for another, lighter one, but I did not expect any complications.

'In four weeks' time he will be as good as new,' were my parting words to the anxious and repentant mother. It was obvious to me that she was suffering terrible remorse for her behaviour that morning.

I was right to say and to think that no further complications would arise and Simon's arm would heal well and soon. I was right about that, but I was very wrong about his mother's unexpected complication.

It was about three or four days later that I received another telephone summons from Anne. It was not as insistent as the first call, but it was professional just the same.

From the moment the caller announced herself, I thought that Simon must have done something he should not, and either broken the plaster or he was having unexpected pain and discomfort – things that can happen in cases such as his.

But no, it wasn't about the boy. Anne was calling me about herself. She was ill with some kind of infection that was causing her a great deal of discomfort. She could not tell me more and I decided to pay her a house visit and see for myself. I told her that I would come that afternoon about three o'clock. The call came about eleven in the morning.

I saw for myself Anne's illness. And what I saw I could hardly believe.

That 'infection', as she called it, had begun on the night following Simon's provoked accident.

About three or four o'clock in the morning she had been awakened by a sudden intensive itching and burning of her right hand and arm. She took some pills to soothe her, bathed the arm in cold water but it did not help. As a matter of fact, it had steadily progressed until it became so unbearable and uncomfortable that she decided to call on me.

When I asked her why did she not call me immediately the following day her answer was that she thought it would pass on its own.

It took me only a few moments to diagnose her condition. Unbelievable as it seemed, (or was it just coincidental?) Anne was suffering from an acute skin infection or better, affliction, that had all the symptoms of severe dermatitis.

When I asked her whether she had had similar skin eruptions in the past, the answer was negative. So were the answers to my questions whether she had used some new detergents, or new creams, eaten exotic food, that could have provoked contact or food dermatitis. I suggested we had better consult my old friend the dermatologist. She consented eagerly because she could no longer endure the itching and pain in her arm, apart from the 'disgusting aspect' as she put it.

The dermatologist confirmed my suspicion of a rather virulent form of dermatitis. Her whole right arm, from the finger tips right up to her shoulder, was affected with blisters and sores. The strange and unusual thing was that it was only on her right arm.

'That's a very unusual case,' the dermatologist told me. 'I've never seen unilateral dermatitis. As a rule, both hands, or arms are affected, seldom, if ever, only one of them,' he explained to us. 'Still, dermatitis is such a peculiar disease and its cause still not known, that one can expect anything, literally anything. As you know,' he turned towards me, 'hereditary factors can play a very important part in its etiology, yet the actual pattern of inheritance is still not well defined. We know of cases where sudden emotion, mental tension, great stress, can trigger off an acute dermatitis.'

'I know, I know,' came the agonising voice of the stricken woman. 'It's my punishment. God is punishing me for being so beastly and cruel to my little boy.' She started to cry. 'I deserve it, more than deserve this punishment for causing my boy to suffer unjustly.'

'Anne, please don't blame yourself,' I tried to calm the distraught woman, who I feared was on the point of becoming hysterical. 'Calm yourself, and don't talk such nonsense.' I tried to be crude. 'How can you blame this illness of yours on what you did to Simon? You didn't break his arm. It was an unfortunate accident, I admit, but to think that you are being punished for that is more than absurd. It's an unfortunate coincidence that has nothing to do with Simon's breaking his arm.'

'It's nice of you to try to comfort me,' she smiled forcedly. 'But I feel it in my soul that this is my punishment and I will not get rid of it as long as I live.'

The dermatologist also said that there could be no connection and suggested that trying to cure the dermatitis was a more practical approach. 'Blaming yourself will do no good to anyone.'

Anne did have treatment for her acute dermatitis. Not one but practically all the known remedies for the cure of skin afflictions were tried out one after the other. Some helped a little for a while. Then the disease would return anew and another remedy would be applied.

Ointments, tar-baths, creams and powders all went the same way. Limited improvement of the itching sensation, less prominent blisters and sores, but it did not clear up completely.

The last flare up came after the day I changed Simon's plaster bandage. Again the mother insisted on being present and she saw the scaly skin of her boy's arm when it was out of the plaster. Scaliness is always a result when a limb is bandaged in plaster for some considerable period of time. I told her this, when I saw she was getting upset by the look of her boy's arm.

I applied another, lighter bandage and the X-ray revealed normal healing of the fractured bone. As I have mentioned, the following day Anne's arm became worse and we were forced once again to change the treatment.

We began seriously to worry about her general condition of health. I even suggested hospitalisation.

Six weeks following Simon's accident, I removed the final plaster of Paris bandage from his arm and after examination he was told that his arm was now as good as it was before, and that he could return to his usual sporting activities.

'Even football and rugby, Simon,' I smiled at the happy boy and sent him into the outstretched arms of his mother.

No, Anne's dermatitis did not disappear immediately following the mending of Simon's arm fracture. It took a few weeks for the dermatitis to disappear completely. But from the day that her boy ceased to be a patient and resumed his usual boisterous activities both at school and at home, her arm began to heal.

It was a slow gradual healing, but the same remedies which before were of no help began to influence the healing process. The blisters disappeared and the itching subsided.

By the time that she had begun to adjust herself to put up with the dermatitis, the final cure began. The skin of her right arm cleared of all blisters and sores; her movement of the arm which was very weak and painful returned to its normal self. It looked as normal as before the first symptoms appeared. And four weeks later both the dermatologist and I could declare her cured and told her that she could discontinue all treatments.

'Will it come again?' she asked, turning towards the specialist.

'Not unless your boy breaks another arm or leg,' he tried to be funny.

But I saw that his joke was not as funny as he pretended it to be. As for myself, I cannot say one way or another. Who knows, perhaps God or some other upholder of justice did punish her for accusing the boy of a crime he did not commit, and punish him at that.

It will remain a mystery for me as long as I go on practising medicine. Perhaps there is some Greater Force above us that guides our destiny!

VIII

Mother Love and a Dying Boy

The tale of Samuel Lyndon Washington Jones is unique for a host of reasons. Had I not been the surgeon on the case, but had merely been told of his injuries, I fear that I should have refused point-blank to credit that any human being could survive this onslaught – no matter what his stamina! Not to speak of the numerous major operations he underwent and braved courageously. Yet in this case I had been the surgeon; there was no question of disbelieving what I myself had performed and witnessed!

In spite of the terrible misfortune which had so cruelly singled him out, Sam, as we all came to call him, was blessed with one supreme advantage! He had at least been born into the twentieth century. For only in this present age is there such an abundance of first-rate surgical means at hand, able to be called upon without delay.

In telling the story of this modern miracle, I must not omit mention of the part so touchingly played by his mother.

I cannot describe her, for any description of mine would most certainly stray grossly from the truth. I cannot describe her face because, to me, hers was a beauty of the spirit that only a Leonardo da Vinci or someone with equally sublime talent could portray.

Hers was probably the most beautiful face I was ever to encounter; and yet let me admit that I never actually saw her face at all! Looking at her, I saw only what she stood for – what she personified – and therefore I found her beautiful. That she was a coffee-skinned, middle-aged negress with thick lips, broad nose and crinkly hair, I knew, but did not see!

If ever a woman stood for all that was civilized and naturally good and gracious, it was this little coloured saint. If ever a woman could lay bare the cruel sinfulness of colour prejudice – again it was the humble Mrs Leona Jones. A purer heart will never beat beneath the most rosy-hued chest!

There she was, either squatting or kneeling by Sam's bed, her eyes seeing what none of us were able to see, riveted not on the mortally-sick youth at her side but on some image that belonged to her alone. Her hands she kept constantly folded over her breast. She was obviously in prayer, yet so modestly and inconspicuously as not to be obtrusive.

Whatever modern surgery and our endeavour did for the body of Samuel Lyndon Washington Jones, his mother's fervent belief and unconquerable trust in God must have done a hundredfold more for his soul. The actual battle for Sam's life had already begun on that Sunday afternoon when, on surveying the twenty-nine injured men, I had to decide dispassionately, on their order of precedence.

Each, of course, desperately needed help and each was to receive it. Deciding which victim could stand waiting for his operation just that little while longer than his neighbour – this was, in itself, a hateful task for a surgeon. Above all, it was a demanding, serious task!

In all honesty, from the seriousness of his injuries, Sam should have been the first. Yet I left him to the very last! At first glance this will undoubtedly appear a most illogical decision, but experience has taught me that it was the only correct one.

The damage to his body was so grave as to make it clear to me that, instead of adding to his chances, immediate surgery might actually cut off altogether these same terribly slender chances of survival.

Any operation, no matter how slight, is in itself a momentary injury to the body of the patient. It produces a state known as surgical shock. In this case, surgical shock added to the shock already received from his other injuries would have been quite beyond even Sam's powers of endurance.

'No,' I had decided. 'This patient cannot be operated on

now!' If he should be dying, why add to his torture? Yet if a faint spark of life still persisted, I would have to feed this spark – and feed it by other means than instant surgery. That is why Sam became the last of my twenty-nine patients – instead of the first one, as would have been his right!

On his arrival at the hospital the young negro was unconscious. The first step, therefore, was to dress his superficial wounds gently; make him as comfortable in bed as possible and sustain and kindle that infinitessimal spark of life still within him.

During the thirty-six hours which to me had spelt interminable work on the other patients, Sam was constantly being administered blood transfusions and oxygen, as well as being injected with heart stimulants.

Sometime during the Monday, the ward sister came to inform me that Jones had regained consciousness. 'He looks a little better, I think, Dr Sava.'

'Really, sister, – why, that's splendid.'

My interest immediately aroused, I rushed between operations down to his ward. I examined him to find out for myself whether the sister's impression had merely been wishful thinking.

But no, she had not imagined things! Sam's condition was definitely showing signs of improvement; however minute these signs, nevertheless he was improving! Only now could I permit myself to examine him, in the certain knowledge that this would not further endanger his condition. On the whole, however, the examination did little to help raise my spirits.

Quite apart from the multiple cuts and bruises, I must own that I felt choking despair at the sight of his mutilated limbs. His left leg was practically torn to pieces – the ankle almost entirely severed, the ends of the broken bones protruding from the wound. Both bones of the leg were fractured; equally so the thigh.

The other leg too, was broken in two places. I gave instructions for the blood transfusion to be continued and prescribed antibiotics. What a battle this would be! I could only be thankful, though, that there still was a battle to be fought.

As I turned to go, I perceived for the first time the tiny, bent figure pathetically hunched in the corner by the top of Sam's bed. A figure which was to become as familiar to me as the sight of the sick man himself. A vision I was to see each and every day and night, throughout the time of our frantic struggle for the youth's life.

Her eyes seemed barely aware of my own or anyone else's presence. When they did shift, it was to settle for a brief moment on the face of the sick boy. So gentle and tender was this glance at her son, so touching in its profound love, that it forced a lump to my throat. It was as if she feared that even a look of less lightness might hurt the outrageously punished body of her boy.

'You are Mrs Jones – Sam's mother?' I whispered softly.

Startled from her reveries, her eyes gradually wandered towards mine as she rose.

'Yes, doctor, I'm Sam's mother.' Those unfathomable eyes still upon mine, she pleaded more than asked: 'Will Sam – he will live, won't he?' After a slight pause she added:

'He's my only child – the best a mother ever had!' This was not said dramatically; just a simple, honest statement.

What was I to reply?

'We're trying very hard,' I told her. 'We're doing all we can – you do know, Mrs Jones!'

'I know it – and may God bless you for it! Doctor, could I – may I stay here with him? I promise I won't disturb him or anyone; I – I just want to be here with him!'

'I'm sure no one will object. You may stay here if you like, only do make sure you get some rest yourself. Will you promise me that?'

'I promise you, doctor, and thank you very much.'

She had not even mentioned her purpose for staying by Sam's bed – so private and personal was her contact with God.

In the course of Monday night Sam's condition continued its slow, steady progress. When I examined him once more on the Tuesday, I felt that delay was no longer advisable. It was now that we had to begin with the operations.

Samuel Lyndon Washington Jones – victim number

twenty-nine on my list of that never-to-be-forgotten holocaust – was wheeled into the operating theatre. For nearly six hours he was under the knife!

First the broken, lacerated ankle was set, reconstructed and sutured. Then came the fracture of the leg; then the thigh. All these fractures had to be reduced by the open method: cutting through the flesh, isolating the bones and fixing the broken ends with metal plates and screws. At last work on the left leg was completed and we could concentrate on the right one. Painstakingly we reconstructed the torn muscles; but not before applying plates and screws once again to the fractured thigh. Both legs were now immobilized in a cast of plaster of Paris. I then called for the X-ray technician and asked for a control examination.

As if guided by some unknown power, I mentioned to the radiologist that I would also like Sam's chest X-rayed. Actually there was no apparent reason for my request. For it was the one part which betrayed no external signs of bruising or injury. So I would have been justified if, for the time being, I had chosen to ignore this part of his anatomy.

Yet, subconsciously, I simply could not credit how with a body as damaged as Sam's, his chest should be let off without a scratch; the obvious, because of its lack of complication, seemed incredible! Whatever my motive – the fact remains that I asked for an immediate chest X-ray on Sam.

When the plates were returned to the theatre and I scrutinized them under the lighted screen I almost broke out in a cold sweat!

'Oh God!' I exclaimed in my horror. Both my assistant and the anaesthetist moved over to me and looked at the plates. Both were soon to draw back aghast, filled with the same emotion as I.

What we saw would have a discouraged a man a great deal more stout-hearted than myself. For it was all there – utter collapse of the left lung with a portion of the diaphragm torn asunder! The chest cavity itself was filled with the organs of the abdomen. This must have resulted from a sudden immense pressure upon the abdomen, thus forcing the organs of the abdomen into the chest.

'It doesn't seem possible!' my assistant muttered. 'How can he possibly still be alive? What in God's name is keeping him alive, George?'

'It's as much of a riddle to me as it is to you.' I had to admit. 'How little we still know of the mysteries of human existence!'

'But – he must die – can you see any other way out?'

'I looked at my assistant for an instant, before I said: 'Operate, doctor!'

He shook his head in doubt. 'Surely he can't stand any more punishment! An operation of this sort would be certain to kill him.' And as if hoping for contradiction, he added: 'Wouldn't it?'

I looked once more at the plates still held clasped in my hands. 'It might – it well might, doctor! But with this boy there's no telling! From what I've seen of his stamina for the last two days, nothing, and I mean literally nothing, would surprise me.'

Still engrossed in the plates, I now stated: 'We're going to try – we're operating! We have nothing to lose; he is going to die, anyway, if we don't operate!' The assistant and the anaesthetist met my eyes in silence, then nodded.

It was, of course, out of the question to follow with a chest operation immediately after the six hours' ordeal Sam had just been subjected to. I therefore ordered him to be taken back to his bed and for his routine treatment to be resumed.

That night, nothing could have dragged me away from the hospital. I had to be near Sam, had to be at hand should his condition deteriorate. What measures, in truth, I could or would have taken, I cannot think! I knew only that I wanted to be there – I knew also that sleep that night at home was out of the question.

There was, however, little change in Sam's condition during the night. Every time I tiptoed up to his bed his mother was there beside him, and I knew that she was praying. Somehow, whenever I came into her vicinity I felt a strange comfort surge through my being. Cynics may scoff; I myself might scoff in my more frivolous moments – yet what I felt then I cannot refute.

Several untouched cups of coffee stood on the little bedside table. I do not recall ever having seen any food pass her lips. Though she remained motionless as a statue, one nevertheless felt her presence strongly. Once I did notice how she stretched out a hand and fleetingly touched the brow of the lad. For a split-second only – as if to reassure herself that life was still there!

Wednesday morning – and Sam was on the operating table once again. He still had difficulty in breathing and had not yet fully regained consciousness from the previous operation.

Before making the final preparations for this fateful intervention I somehow felt the urge to speak to Mrs Jones. I told myself it was to calm and console her; more likely, as I now believe, it was to become infected with a little of her own quiet courage.

This time, as soon as she saw me, she rose and came towards me. If anything, she was even more tranquil and serene that morning. It was she who now addressed me.

'You're going to operate again, aren't you, doctor?' she whispered in her lilting, soft Southern drawl.

'Yes, my dear, we must. We discovered yesterday that Sam's chest is badly hurt, too.'

She merely nodded – nothing could shock or unbalance her by now. 'God will guide you, doctor, to save my boy's life – I know it.'

How beautiful this woman was! Her acceptance of any situation, her trust and confidence – they were infectious. Suddenly I, too, felt that the final outcome of Sam's struggle might really be a happy one; suddenly I felt easier, less heavy-hearted at the difficult task ahead of me.

I took the small hand in mine and pressed it for a moment. 'I'm truly glad you feel this way, Mrs Jones.' Then, with one last glance at her face – the face I was never to see – I walked away to commence work on the body of her son.

It was thoracic surgery that was called for now. I had no cause to fear any unforeseen complications; whatever I might encounter after opening the chest, I was certain I would be able to cope with it.

The chest was opened through the seventh intercostal space – this meant cutting between the seventh and eighth ribs. Once inside, my hands tried to unravel the coils of intestine and stomach that had become so dislodged from their normal position in the abdomen.

Gradually, the organs were unwound and pushed back through the opening of the lacerated diaphragm into the abdominal cavity. To facilitate this task, a rubber tube was inserted through the mouth into the stomach, so that we might be able to aspirate all the contents of stomach and intestines.

This done satisfactorily, we now had to reconstruct the torn diaphragm – in itself no trivial undertaking. Piece by piece the fragments of the diaphragm were brought together and joined one to another by means of cat-gut stitches.

Three hours had already elapsed. Not infrequently, I stole furtive glances at the anaesthetist who again had taken on the charge of seeing that Sam received as little as possible of the anaesthetics.

Quite frankly I dreaded asking him outright about the patient's condition. Any doubtful, let alone discouraging reply now, I feared, might wipe out my confidence. Sam was still breathing – that much I knew! How precarious his condition might have become I preferred not to know just then. At any rate, I had no choice now; I had to finish what I had set out to do.

The end of the operation was at last in sight. I assured and reassured myself that there was no bleeding and that all the organs were in their correct positions. Then I asked the anaesthetist to force air into the collapsed left lung.

What satisfaction to watch while the small dark piece of flesh – all that the lung had become – began gradually to expand and to creep stealthily forward, a creature with a life of its own! The dark colour soon retreated until it faded entirely to give place to a soft, pink hue. I touched the lung gently.

'No more shocks!' I pleaded silently. 'Please God, just no more new complications!'

The lung itself, however, was healthy. No injury of any kind made itself apparent. So its collapse had obviously been caused only by the invasion of the abdominal intruders!

'Thank God!' I muttered again. 'Thank God!'

What now remained to be done was to bring the divided ribs together and to unite once again into one whole the separated muscles and skin of the chest.

A small rubber drain was placed inside the chest cavity and fastened trimly to the edge of the wound. Later, once the patient was safely back in bed, it would be connected to a suction machine. This would ensure that no fluid could collect in the chest-cavity. Were this to happen it might result in the lung's collapsing for a second time.

The fight for Sam's life still raged tense and fierce! Only now we were no longer on the defensive, we had become the stronger opponent – the attackers!

Sam was alive and Sam was to remain alive. His bones were to mend: slowly, gradually, bone by broken bone. His wounds were to heal and his bruised flesh was in time to become normal. Death had fumed and snorted, bent on prematurely pilfering the young negro's life. Yet death had been beaten down out of sight – to spit her cruel curses elsewhere!

We had all had our various small parts to perform in this victory. The nurses had given unstinted, endless service, comfort and understanding. The surgical assistant, untiring at all times of day and night, had been at the ready with blood transfusions and injections. The anaesthesia was never anything but outstanding. And I suppose Tom's, Dick's and Harry's techniques in abdominal, thoracic and orthopaedic surgery had played their part! Thank heaven that I had at least been capable of making fair use of their teaching; for I had combined my own European training with the best of what I had gleaned in America. It was this which had constituted the surgery performed on Samuel Lyndon Washington Jones!

Yet to my mind the strongest crusader, the real victor, was the most silent, least assertive member of our small army – that fragile, quiet figure at Sam's bedside, that frail black woman with the staunch courage of the early martyrs!

Much as I advocate and believe in practical aid, nothing will ever convince me that it was not that mother's prayers which saved her son above everything else. That it was not her faith which moved the Almighty to hear and answer.

IX

Prayers and Abortion

My first involvement with positive thinking and prayers as opposed to suggest abortion in order to avoid the birth of a deformed child came when I met Valerie at my consulting rooms in London

I had known Valerie and her husband for a long time, but only as friends. Many times we had partnered each other at the tennis club of which we were members. It was there that Valerie met her future husband.

Often in those vivid recalled days before I decided to leave for Australia, following my car accident – they seem to belong to a different age – I always marvelled at how happily and ideally matched they were. It was not merely that they were both physically attractive and pleasant people. They seemed, at any rate to an outsider, to have many interests in common.

It was just before I received an invitation to come to Australia to recover from the accident and three years after their marriage on which occasion too, I was present. But after that I was so immersed in work that for a while I completely lost sight of them, though news of them would reach me on occasions. And what I heard confirmed all my early impressions.

They were the perfectly married couple – a rare occasion in these days of easy divorce. But what a pity it was, some friends remarked, that they still had no family now that they had celebrated their fourth anniversary.

It was exactly the day after their fourth anniversary that Valerie came to see me professionally. Apart from the trickle of gossip that had reached me I knew practically nothing about her problems, but I really felt happy to renew our once warm friendship. It was on spotting her name on my waiting list that old, sweet memories of our relationship were once more conjured up. She had appointed the hour for her visit so unusually late that I concluded it was of a personal and not a professional nature.

'It's lovely to see you again, Valerie,' I said, as she was shown into my room. 'I forget how long it is since we last met, but in any case it's far too long. I hope you've come for a friendly chat and not as a patient seeking medical advice.' But even as I said these words I felt their emptiness.

Valerie looked anxious and distraught. 'How's Bob?' I added hastily, hoping to bring the subject on safer, more familiar ground.

'Oh, he's fine, always busy in his new job,' she replied, and began explaining what her husband's new job was. 'But I have come to see you, George, partly as a friend and partly as a doctor, I mean, I want to consult you because I believe that, since we are also friends, you will tell me the truth. That sounds like an awful cliché, doesn't it?' She made an effort to smile brightly. 'But I think you understand what I mean.'

'I think I can guess,' I replied. 'You look worried, Valerie. What's the trouble?' I began to suspect that it was some problem in her marriage she had come to discuss with a friend.

'Well ....' She hesitated, appearing suddenly bashful. An unusual thing for her.

Valerie was not a bold woman, but was always frank and open, and this reluctance to speak helped to confirm my suspicions that it was more a domestic than a medical problem she had come to discuss.

'It's like this,' she went on slowly. 'No two people could be happier together than Bob and I. It's wonderful,' she said, and the glow in her eyes could only confirm her sincerity. 'But – well, there's one thing that rather casts a shadow over our lives. You see, both of us are desperately keen to have children, and though we've tried and tried – well, nothing has happened so far. And that's four years of trying!'

'Well, it's nice to know that you, at least, are not one of

those couples who tend to avoid having children at all costs,' I joked inanely. 'In what way can I be of help?'

I spoke more as friend than a doctor. It was best to keep the tone of the conversation light under the circumstances.

'I really don't know,' she said with a worried frown. 'You see, as soon as we realised our efforts were unsuccessful, we naturally suspected that one or other of us must have something defective. So I went to our family doctor. He's a nice old boy, though he is getting a bit doddery. He's almost on the point of retiring, but he still knows more than enough.'

'Well?'

'What he eventually told me,' she continued in a sad voice, her head bent, 'shocked us both terribly. He said it would be impossible for me to have a child!'

'What?' I sat up sharply. 'Did he tell you why?'

She nodded. 'Yes. He said I wasn't properly developed or something like that.'

I frowned. This was indeed a very rash statement on the face of it. Valerie was, to all outward appearances, a thoroughly normal young woman; and it is part of every normal woman's make-up to be able to bear children.

I thought of the mental picture her description of her GP had conjured up: old, doddery, and on the point of retiring. Probably he didn't want to know of modern advances in the diagnosis and treatment of infertility.

'That is certainly a rash statement,' I remarked. 'Did he examine you?'

'Well yes. And he asked a lot of questions about my menstrual periods, and then said: "I'm afraid there's only one conclusion to arrive at – you've an infertile uterus and you'll be unable to conceive." And so that was that.'

'I presume then, that you've come to me for a different opinion – if possible?'

'Oh, yes. Bob also thought it would be a good idea, because in you we don't just have a fine doctor but a friend. If our old doctor is really right, then we shall have to face it and give up the idea, though that would be as big a blow to Bob as it would to me. But if there is some hope ... Well, both of us are ready to face any reasonable risk.'

'I can't give you my opinion off-hand. I know nothing about you medically. It's been years. You'd better come along tomorrow to the hospital where I can have you examined thoroughly. But you can take it from me that young women aren't sterile for no apparent reason. There must be some definite cause for it. An infantile uterus is, admittedly, one of them. But to state a cause just from a perfunctory examination is a rash deduction. I'm afraid you have to go through a lengthy examination and if we can discover that cause we may be able to do something about it. Even an infantile uterus can be made to become fertile, you know ...'

'Oh, I hope so, George, I really hope so!' Her voice was tremulous. 'That gives me hope, at least. It seems so unfair. After all, I've been so fit all my life.'

'Quite.' I nodded emphatically. 'And for that reason you must not despair, my dear. First let us find out the real cause for your inability to conceive.'

'Thank you, George,' she said in a husky voice. 'Thank you with all my heart.'

A little later Valerie left my rooms and I began to speculate on the subject. The more I thought about it, the more ridiculous the situation appeared to me. This doctor, after a brief examination, and few hasty questions, had arrived at a sweeping, dogmatic conclusion that could be ascertained only through the most searching investigation. More than that, he took for granted that, if sterility existed, it lay in Valerie herself and quite ignored the fact that, in modern civilisation sterility is at least as common in men as in women; indeed, there is something more than a suggestion that it is more prevalent in men.

I was annoyed at this dictum, not merely because it was casual and unscientific, but because it had been given in such a way as to cause mental distress to the patient. Its finality, too, was another thing that was insufferable. And the majority of women would probably have accepted this opinion as final and not taken even the precaution of seeking another and perhaps more expert opinion.

My doubts swelled at the first examination. So far as the most rigorous external examination could reveal Valerie was a perfectly healthy, normal woman, with a strong desire for motherhood. There was nothing at all on which to base even the tentative diagnosis of an infantile uterus. What then, was wrong?

The only way to discover that, I decided, was to make an exploratory abdominal examination. There was a simple, straightforward way of doing this – a laparoscopy. Through a minute incision just below the navel, a specially designed instrument with a light bulb on its end – like a torch – is introduced into the abdominal cavity after some air is pumped into the abdomen to avoid injuries of the intestines. This enables one to inspect with precision all the abdominal organs and find out if anything is wrong with one or other of them. The uterus is particularly easily examined in this fashion, thus avoiding the more dangerous and lengthier explorative operation.

I explained all this to Valerie and she acquiesced readily. Indeed she welcomed it. She felt, I think, that this at least would decide the matter. It was taking the case to the last court of appeal, and if the verdict were negative then it would have to be accepted for what it was. But at least, there would be no torturing doubts left.

At her own insistence I did the laparoscopy myself. I was determined to do my best for her. She had suffered enough already – first from the thwarting of her hopes, and then from the rebuff she had received when, like a prudent person, she had sought advice.

In due course Valerie was admitted to the hospital, and I performed the laparoscopy. Debating with myself over the case, several possibilities had occurred to me, and I had passed everything in review. But I was not fully prepared for what I did in fact discover.

There was a small growth at the apex of the womb, no bigger than a walnut and not in itself ominous. But it was sufficient to block the fallopian tubes of the womb, thus preventing the eggs from the ovaries from reaching the inside of the uterus. Everything else appeared normal. It was obvious to me that an operation was necessary to remove the growth.

As Valerie had given her signed permission for me to do

what I considered necessary, there was no problem in changing the procedure. I managed to excise the tumour and free the tube openings in the uterus. The operation took slightly over one hour.

Valerie's subsequent recovery was perfectly normal. Her condition never gave me the slightest anxiety; in fact, she revealed a degree of physical stamina beyond even what might have been expected from a young woman in normal health.

When two months later, news reached me that she was pregnant, I felt that final glow of satisfaction that comes when an ambition is realised. Once more she came to me for advice.

She was by then in her second month of pregnancy, but had come to consult me about a rash that had broken out all over her body. She told me that for the last three days she was running a temperature but felt fine otherwise.

A sudden fear gripped me. 'Let's look at the rash, Valerie,' I said gingerly. She took off her blouse and I examined her chest. My heart sank.

'Have you been in contact with friends who have children?' I asked.

'Yes, our neighbours. They have two lovely children who have just recovered from a bout of measles.'

'My God!' I exclaimed. 'Valerie, I'm afraid you have measles! But we must make sure.'

I arranged at once for her to consult a specialist. There be no more speculating when the answer came. Valerie had measles and she was two months pregnant!

How could fate be this cruel? Valerie had sacrified everything for the coming baby. It was not certain that she could have another if this one was aborted. How could I tell her, if indeed she did not know it herself full-well, that expectant mothers who contract measles in the first two or three months of pregnancy are in danger of giving birth to deformed or mentally deficient babies. It is an accepted medical dictum that in such cases it is advisable to terminate the pregnancy.

The specialist was of the opinion that the pregnancy must be terminated as soon as possible. Prevarication could prove dangerous for the mother herself. I braced myself for a confrontation with Valerie and her husband.

And when they came to see me again I told them as gently as I could that it would be necessary to terminate the pregnancy because of the high risk to the baby. 'Surely you wouldn't take that risk?' I asked more as a formality, certain that she would refuse.

And yet, I'm still not quite sure why, but while waiting for the couple, I had begun to have doubts about the inevitablity of terminating the pregnancy. After all the suffering Valerie had gone through. After all these wild expectations of a new mother. My heart went out to Valerie as I watched her weeping in silence as I pointed out all the perils of her condition.

Her husband held her hand without saying a word. In his eyes I read only despair. 'It isn't fair,' he said at length. 'Val doesn't deserve such punishment!' Valerie continued to weep silently, all her sorrow and agony pouring out of her.

I let her cry for a while. It was better so. Then looking at her and sensing her desperation. I decided to act as I had never acted before. If she decided to carry on with her pregnancy in spite of all the dangers – I would support her instead of insisting on an abortion. But I was going to wait and see what her own intentions were.

All at once her face lit up as she raised her head and looked me straight in the eyes,

'George,' she began, 'I don't know what you will say – but I've decided not to have an abortion! This is my last – my only chance to have a child. No, no abortion! I'm going to have that baby no matter how it turns out. I would rather look after a deformed baby than no baby. If God has decided that my baby will be deformed, so be it. Then I will simply devote my whole life to it.'

'Thank God,' I mumbled. I smiled at her and took her free hand in mine. 'I'm glad, Valerie that you have decided to keep the baby,' I said, to her surprise.

'Do you mean that?' She almost fell into my arms as she rose and came towards me. 'I thought you would insist on an abortion.'

'Yes,' I confessed. 'All my training and experience, my so-called duty as a physician would point to that. But, deep in my heart I was hoping you would decline to have the pregnancy terminated.'

I paused for a moment. 'I know that I will be criticised severely for taking that attitude by many of my colleagues. But I speak to you as a friend, not as a doctor. You, Valerie, have your baby!'

Her husband now spoke: 'Darling,' he said. 'Is that your wish? To have the baby no matter what the dangers?'

'Yes,' she said gently but firmly.

'Right, Val,' he grinned at her. 'We'll have our baby and we'll face anything that comes – together.'

Now that a great burden was lifted from me, I decided to act. I told them that they had to think positive. No more doubts as to whether the baby will be deformed. 'From now on, Valerie,' I insisted. 'You will think only good, positive thoughts. You will have a normal baby! You will pray as you have never prayed before that the baby you are carrying in your body will be a lovely, normal little being.'

I held her hand again. 'Promise me that!'

'I promise,' she nodded in understanding. 'I have prayed all these years for a baby and you helped me to have one. Now I shall pray even more strongly that God gives me a healthy baby. He *will* listen to me.'

She spoke with sincerity and genuine hope, not like someone desperate who reaches for the last straw. Valerie meant what she was saying. I knew that she would take my advice and go on thinking positive; go on praying and looking forward to the arrival of the baby.

We parted on that note and I was left brooding on my unorthodox behaviour. What would my colleagues say when the child was born?

'Just luck, old boy, just luck,' they would concede if the child was normal.

But what would they say if, as was expected by the experts, a deformed baby came into the world? What would their verdict be then? I shuddered to think of all the accusations that would be hurled at me. Yet I simply would not allow myself to be gripped by such thoughts for any length of time.

I, too, was thinking positive. Valerie's baby was going to be a normal little child – charming and strong as its mother.

Valerie came to see me regularly. We saw a gynaecologist who was rather surprised at the attitude we had taken.

'It's a rash decision, my friend,' he said to me in private. 'You must have known the dangers. Measles during the second month of pregnancy is bound to affect the child. It will be a deformed baby, to be sure, if not mentally deficient as well.'

'I know the dangers, and so does the patient,' I replied calmly. 'But she would rather have a deformed baby than no baby at all.'

He remained silent for a moment. Then, as if in afterthought he remarked; 'You know she might well have a difficult delivery. Her pelvis is rather narrow and you say you removed a growth from the apex of her womb?'

'Yes.' And I explained in detail Valerie's infertility and the operation I performed.

'In that case, if she wants to see her baby alive she must have a Caesarian section delivery.'

'Will you perform it?'

'No, if you don't mind,' he said curtly. 'Since I believe strongly that the pregnancy should have been terminated, I do not wish to have anything to do with the case.'

A new problem was now facing me. I had to explain to Valerie the dangers of having a normal delivery.

'You mean the baby might die?' she asked.

'Yes. And your own life might be in danger.'

'What are we to do?'

'I would advise a Caesarian section. You know what that means?'

'Yes. Delivering the baby through my tummy.'

I smiled. 'You're a brave and courageous girl, Valerie. We must find a good gynaecologist who will perform the operation.'

I did not tell her that I had already had one refusal. But I was hoping we would find a man who would have less scruples and more humanity to perform the operation. But here I did not reckon with Valerie's stubbornness.

'No, George,' she answered. We don't need anyone else. You made it possible for me to have this baby. You agreed with me that I should not have an abortion. So, my friend, you will have to deliver the baby. And who knows the inside of my tummy better than you? You've already looked inside once.' She smiled disarmingly at me, showing me that as far as she was concerned the question was settled.

'But, Valerie,' I protested. 'It's a case for a gynaecologist and an obstetrician; it's not my speciality.'

Bob, her husband, made a gesture of annoyance at this point. 'We've had enough of specialists of that kind. George,' he insisted, 'you are the only specialist we need. Both Valerie and I have the utmost faith in you.'

I pondered. It was quite true that this was really outside my practice, yet there were other factors. I still had that feeling of guilt to expunge. After all I had so much at stake. It was a special case for me in more than one sense. In a unique way, it was my own. More than that, this pregnancy was the direct outcome of the operation I had performed. It was also the outcome of the advice I had given to carry on with the pregnancy in direct opposition to that given by the majority of my colleagues.

That alone was something I could not shirk. Having given it, in the full knowledge of what I was doing, I could hardly at this stage, when it had been acted upon, try to shift the burden on to someone else – even if I could find someone.

'Very well,' I said, though making no effort to hide my reluctance. 'I will operate on Valerie when the time comes, if that is what you both wish.'

'Thank you again, George,' Valerie beamed. 'You've taken a load off our minds.'

Two weeks before the full term of pregnancy, I performed the Caesarian section. Every moment was tense, but at last it was done. We had succeeded – so far. The baby was a girl.

I had a curious feeling, almost fear, that kept me for a moment from looking and inspecting the newly-born baby. Then, as if from afar, came the voice of the nurse:

'What a beautiful baby, doctor!'

At that moment I turned my head towards the nurse who was studying the baby rapturously. A piercing cry at that instant informed us that the newcomer also had strong lungs.

It was a reward not given often to a man. But it was Valerie's positive thinking and implicit trust in God which really brought that healthy baby into the world ...

When I left the hospital I was still filled with doubts. There were anxious moments still to pass. The baby looked normal physically. But what about her mental state? That would be shown in later days as the child grew older.

But for the moment it seemed fate was smiling on Valerie. Both she and the baby were in good shape when I visited them the next morning.

During the night I had certainly expected to be woken by the phone. But that night it did not ring. The last report I had had was that everything was satisfactory.

I set out early for the hospital and I was somewhat alarmed when the Matron asked me to go at once to Valerie's room. Had some sudden crisis developed after all, then?

'I think you should see her now,' the matron said ambiguously.

I braced myself for a shock. And I did, indeed, experience shock but it was not at all what I had feared.

Not merely was Valerie in fine fettle; she was actually sitting up in bed and eating her breakfast. On a chair, gazing at her with adoring eyes, was Bob, her husband. His glance passed to me dumbly, as though joy and relief had robbed him of all powers of speech. And then, slowly, like a man in a dream he rose and held out his hand.

This simple, warm gesture was more eloquent even than the torrent of phrases of gratitude.

'We can never thank you enough, George,' they both insisted time and again.

'Rubbish!' I replied. 'I have to thank you both for your trust, and your unswerving belief in God's goodness. You've behaved admirably, Valerie. You're the real heroine of this story. It needed courage to run the risk you did. It's all turned out well, but it could just as easily have turned to tragedy.

Perhaps even more easily.' I added aside.

'I didn't have the slightest doubt that everything would turn out well. And you, my friend, with your insistence on positive thought made me determined and gave me the courage to go on with my pregnancy.'

Her face had a serenity, a beauty of fulfilment in it that was a joy to behold.

Yes, it might easily have been a tragedy – a deeper tragedy even than having a deformed baby. For it had been a bold decision on my part; a decision against all my earlier principles.

If I had been wise and spoken according to the book of caution, I should never have allowed the pregnancy to continue undisturbed. But I could not find the courage nor the temerity to kill the one desire that kept Valerie alive. Her unborn baby!

I sensed that not only their marriage, but Valerie's entire existence was at stake here. So, I transgressed all the laws of medicine and encouraged her to go on with her pregnancy.

There are things not mentioned in the bulky tomes that line my reference bookshelves. They can tell me all I may want to know about this and that disease; about how authorities regard abortion as the only treatment in women who have contracted measles during their early pregnancies. But they never talk of joy and happiness.

Surgeons, faced with facts, tend to forget those things. Yet can there be life without them? Is life without them really life? There are people who would take any risk for complete happiness, yet would not move an inch merely to ensure the continuity of mere existence. The surgeons, too, must be on the side of the angels sometimes.

And that reminds me that my friends christened their baby Angela. I was present at the ceremony, for I had been asked to be godfather.

This child, in a very special sense, was mine to sponsor. If I looked at it with pride and thankfulness, that was as nothing to the ecstatic glow on the faces of her parents.

In preventing this life from being extinguished and instead

bringing it safely into the world, I had made an entity of three.

Soon after Angela's christening I had my car accident which so very nearly extinguished my own life. Perhaps by bringing Angela into the world I had made a contribution for which God decided I should live.

X

Love a Duck

It had been a glorious month – my first month in Perth. At last I was fulfilling a life-time dream to live in Australia and explore its beauties.

As I did not have too many patients during that month, I decided to fulfil another dream of mine – to see or work as a Flying Doctor. I wrote to a friend of mine who was in charge of one of the West Australia stations. I asked him whether he knew of a vacancy in their service. I told him that I had started practice in Perth, but not being busy I would like to locum for some Flying Doctor who needed a vacation.

The reply was immediate. Not only he said were there many vacancies, but he himself was in need of a substitute. Could I come as soon as possible.

And so it was that I found myself working as 'Flying Locum' at the station where my friend Dr Harvey James conducted his clinic on the air.

Although in general all base hospitals were run on similiar lines, each one had its own routine, its own little laws, its own peculiarities. So I was very grateful to Harvey James for letting me come two days before he actually left. I had the opportunity of watching the master at work.

One of the laws of the Flying Doctor Service, unwritten but none-the-less strictly adhered to, was that no patient could interrupt a consultation between a doctor and his distant patient, unless it was a real emergency.

It was my second day at the new base hospital, and the air clinic had just begun.

I saw Dr Harvey James was already in consultation. It was

eight o'clock, the hour I was told the work started. But a little later I was to discover that one of Harvey's idiosyncrasies was his idea of punctuality. It seemed that when he said eight o'clock he meant ten minutes to eight and no matter what time he might mention for an appointment – he always meant ten minutes earlier.

'Good morning, Dr James. S for sugar here. How are you? Over!'

Harvey smiled softly.

'Good morning, Mrs Cooper. I'm fine. Anything the matter with you?"

'No, not me, doctor. It's Robbie again. He's in bed with an upset stomach. Over!'

'Mm. Now let me see – when was it we took his appendix out?'

'About three weeks ago, doctor.' This from the nurse who like myself was listening in to every consultation.

'Oh yes, three weeks. Have you been feeding him too well again, Mrs Cooper?'

'No, doctor, not me. But you know yourself what he's like. Every time he comes in the house it's straight to the pantry.'

'Yes, I know, little Robbie likes his food. It sounds like a case of indigestion, Mrs Cooper. Just give him some of that white medicine I left with you.'

'Sure, doctor, thank you. Over!'

A slight pause, no more than a minute or two. Then a new voice came over the air.

'Morning, doctor! This is H for Hobby. Over!'

'Ah, Tim, good morning. How's the leg this morning?'

'Better, doctor. Just want to tell you that the medicine is doing its stuff. My leg is less swollen now.' Tim was an old cobber, and his was one of the first voices I learned to recognize.

'But there's something else –' At that moment there was a sudden blur and Tim's voice was lost. Instead, a new voice cut in.

'A for Auntie – are you receiving me?' There was anxiety in the voice of the new caller, to be sure, and it was that of an old lady.

'Dear me,' I said to myself, 'this must be serious. It had better be or Harvey will have something to say.'

But somehow Harvey seemed to take this interruption with surprising calm. He and the nurse exchanged quick glances, and both of them smiled broadly. I was puzzled and felt the outsider I was.

'Aunt Penny,' he whispered.

'Tim,' he said into the microphone, 'would you mind? I'll be back with you in a jiffy.'

'Sure, doctor, you take your time,' replied Tim 'you'd better attend to Aunt Penny – sounds as if she's in trouble.'

Harvey returned to A for Auntie.

'Good morning, Aunt Penny. What's wrong?'

'Oh my, doctor, I'm so upset – so worried. Jemima's not eating! She's ailing something terrible!' I began to picture the emergency-caller. An old lady, frail but still full of energy.

As I have already said, Harvey was not in the least put out by this dramatic plea for help. His handsome face was creased in smiles.

'You'll have to have another go at feeding her, Aunt Penny. Just try again.'

'But it's no use,' the old lady replied. 'I've tried near a dozen times, doctor.'

'Mm,' Harvey paused for thought. 'Try stuffing it down her throat.'

'But?'

'Oh come on now, Aunt Penny. You know that in a case like this it pays to be cruel so that you can be kind.'

To be quite frank, by now I was thoroughly confused and not a little taken aback. Obviously the old lady was anxious about a child, perhaps her little grand-daughter. 'Stuffing it down her throat,' forcing a child to eat when it did not feel like eating, struck me as a rather cruel procedure.

'Anyway,' Aunt Penny was saying, 'I've tried stuffing it down her throat but she brought it all up again. What shall I do – just what on earth shall I do?'

'Now, now, Aunt Penny,' said Harvey soothingly, 'just you take it easy. Remember your own heart!'

'But that's what'll break it if we don't get Jemima better,' whimpered the old lady.

'She'll get better all right. You give her those pills I left for her last time.'

'But, doctor, she's so much worse now. She won't even look at the dog. And another thing, remember when Rover bit her leg? Well, it's swollen up again.'

'Mm. She must be feverish then. Better let her have the penicillin tablets – you still have some left?'

'Yes.'

'Good. No more than two at a time twice daily.'

'That's all very well, doctor. But just how do I get her to take them?'

Harvey smiled.

'Oh, Aunt Penny – you've had Jemima all this time now,' he said, 'surely you know what to do?' To my amazement, Harvey sounded neither impatient nor did he seem to be joking.

'Just get a hold of her beak,' he instructed, 'pull it open and push the two tablets down. Then keep it shut for a few minutes.'

If until that moment I was merely puzzled, now I was altogether dazed. I could not bear the suspense any longer. 'Chasing dogs,' 'bitten in the leg,' and now 'stuffing penicillin down her beak!'

'Harvey,' I said at last. 'If I didn't know we were conducting a clinic on the air, I would have thought that I was about to deputise for a veterinary surgeon. Or could it be that some Aborigines have beaks instead of mouths?'

Harvey James roared with laughter.

'Sava,' he beamed, 'what an imagination you have. "Abos" with beaks for mouths! Can you beat that? No, my friend, our Aborigines do not have beaks, I assure you.'

'Then why all these instructions?'

'It just so happened,' he went on, 'that Jemima is a duck – and you will agree that ducks have beaks?'

'A duck?' I exclaimed, 'a duck! And you actually permitted the interruption of a serious consultation because of that duck?'

'George,' he said. 'There's something you should know.

Jemima may be a duck – but not an ordinary one as you may think. She happens to be the duck of the Outback. She enjoys great renown, great respect and great love. I'll tell you all about her later.'

'OK, Aunt Penny,' Harvey returned to his consultation with the owner of Jemima. 'Sorry for the interruption. Here with me is Dr George Sava just arrived from England. Obviously he hasn't heard yet about our Jemima. Anyway, you do as I told you and let me know how you get on.'

'I'll try,' said Aunt Penny, 'and please tell your friend about my Jemima.'

Now that Aunt Penny was off the air Harvey returned to H for Hobby and Tim's bad leg. Then followed a case of whooping cough.

There were many other calls during the two-hour clinic on the air but no more emergency interruptions. All was back to normal – excepting myself. I still had not quite recovered from the shock of the sick duck who took precedence over all the sick 'cobbers', Aborigines and ailing children.

At last it was time for the lunch-break.

And it was then that Harvey told me the story of Jemima the duck and her 'mother' Aunt Penny.

Penny Rafferty and her husband were amongst the original settlers of the Outback. They were an ideal family, proud of each other and happiest when in each other's company. But suddenly all this came to a stop. Tragedy struck.

There were two strong, young sons – Rafferty's only children – who were amongst the first to volunteer when war broke out. They never came back, both being killed in Africa. Old Walter Rafferty followed soon after his sons leaving Penny alone. Everyone expected her to pack up, sell the property and perhaps return to her native Ireland.

But that is where everyone made a mistake. For Aunt Penny simply was not a person about whom any kind of speculation could be made. She stayed right where she was, tending her station, working from dawn to dusk – trying to forget. Her inseparable companions were a huge, shaggy watchdog named Rover and a snow-white pet duck named Jemima.

Undoubtedly pride of place in Penny's affections was held

by the remarkable Jemima. And she was something quite special, something quite unducklike, something few ducks, if any, could ever claim to be.

Jemima was a heroine! What greater heroics can there be than to save a human life? And that is exactly what Jemima had done. She had saved the life of none other than Aunt Penny herself.

Some years ago, Aunt Penny's house caught fire and, if it had not been for Jemima's frantic quacking, Aunt Penny would not be alive today. Nor would Jemima cease quacking until she had made certain she had caught Aunt Penny's ear and woken her from her heavy, working woman's slumber.

Word of Jemima's great deed of heroism soon travelled the length and breadth of the entire area. It became the conversation-piece of the Outback. Aunt Penny would speak for hours of her intelligence, her integrity, her supreme devotion. Yes, Jemima was a duck in a million.

For the next two days I was to witness how beloved was Jemima by all the settlers thereabout. Everyone wanted to know of her progress.

In the mornings, as soon as the air clinic opened, Aunt Penny called to tell us of Jemima's progress. And naturally everyone tuned in to listen. You might almost have called that first quarter of an hour on the air, the 'duck's clinic.'

On the second day of Jemima's illness, Harvey James left for his holidays and it thus fell to me to give further instruction for Jemima's treatment. In no time I became an almost expert veterinarian prescribing pills and potions for other ailing ducks, lame geese and even a coughing cat!

A week later Jemima was cured. Cheerfully chasing Rover, the dog, once again across Aunt Penny's yard and quacking away to her's and Aunt Penny's heart's content.

Yes, Jemima certainly was a duck in a million. Her choice of doctors too could have been a great deal worse. She was the only duck who could claim to have been treated by George Sava come all the way from London's Harley Street!

Aunt Penny was obviously satisfied with my treatment of the patient. And when Aunt Penny actually invited me to visit her and stay for a week-end after my month's work was over, everyone congratulated me.

'You've made the grade, Dr Sava,' they all said. 'Yes, you've certainly made the grade.'

I accepted Aunt Penny's invitation. As soon as Harvey James returned from his vacation, I went to visit Aunt Penny and the renowned Jemima before returning to my practice in Perth. As I drove there I could hear that old cockney phrase: 'Lumme, love a duck!'

Aunt Penny proved to be a delightful old lady with all of the Irish charm, blarney and garrulousness. I took an instant liking to her. More, Aunt Penny was the sort of old lady who would never be old, one whom one simply had to love.

As for Jemima – that duck was a pure gem. As adorable, as 'quackative' a duck as you will ever come across. Her face was remarkably lovely – for a duck's face, at any rate. And when she permitted me to pat her and placed herself comfortably upon my knee, I almost considered getting myself a pet duck too some day. 'She likes you, Dr Sava. Jemima likes you a lot,' Aunt Penny said smiling.

'Well,' I smiled back, 'an intelligent girl like her probably recognises her own doctor. She's grateful and satisfied with her treatment, that's all.'

'I think you're right,' said Aunt Penny solemnly.

Months later, when I was back in London once more, I was to hear the final chapter in the Jemima story.

It appears that some Aborigine was engaged in trapping wild horses. some of the horses strayed right through Aunt Penny's property. Poor Jemima happened to be in the path of one of these wild horses and before she could ever utter a quack, she was trampled to death.

I can well imagine Aunt Penny's grief. That duck had become the joy, the pride of her lonely days. I heard that all who knew Jemima joined in Aunt Penny's sorrow, and many wrote letters of condolence.

With true Australian generosity many sent their own pets to help make Aunt Penny's station more cheerful and alive. And Harvey wrote: 'That yard's brim-full of ducks and geese and what have you, George. You can hear the noise from miles away. It sounds more like a zoo than a station these days.

There are even a couple of mocking birds and cockatoos!'

Aunt Penny, I know, is still at the station, and she still worships ducks. She has quite a number of them now, but not a single one is called Jemima.

For, quite understandably, there will forever be but one Jemima for Aunt Penny – and that unique bird is now lovingly buried in a quiet place at Aunt Penny's station in the Outback.

XI

The Swallowed Teeth

My polite good-bye to my last patient of the day froze on my lips as the telephone rattled its empty head and demanded attention. I said, 'Excuse me,' and picked up the receiver.

'Yes, hello, this is Mr Sava,' I said, emphasizing the 'Mister' and the fact that I was no physician, but a surgeon. 'What can I do for you?'

'I'm Mr Manley – Edward Manley,' said a very agitated voice, also emphasizing his status but making it sufficiently clear that he was in no way connected with my line of business. 'I'm Mr Manley, the husband of Mrs Manley,' he continued, being very revealing.

'Oh yes,' said I, pretending that it was as it should be. 'And ...?'

'Please come over at once. You must. You simply must hurry, doctor,' Mr Manley implored me.

'Please, Mr Manley, tell me what has happened,' I asked, capturing his tearful voice.

'I've sent her to your hospital.'

'Yes, yes, but what has happened?'

'Something dreadful.'

'But what? What?'

'Pardon me, Mrs Sava, I mean Mr Sava – really I don't know what I'm saying. I've only been married for three months and now ...'

I decided to be firm. We were wasting precious minutes. I had to know what was wrong, otherwise I would not know how to function.

'What has happened to your wife?' I shouted abruptly.

'It's her teeth ...'

'I'm not a dentist,' I snapped. 'And please pull yourself together, Mr Manley. What's happened to your wife's teeth?' I already knew the answer intuitively, but I thought it would be better for Edward Manley to corroborate.

'She's swallowed them,' Mr Manley said mournfully. 'The whole top row, and she nearly choked.'

'Good Lord,' I said. 'What did you do?'

'I banged her on the back and she swallowed the plate ... and ...'

There was no more time to be wasted. I managed to get rid of my last patient as politely as I could and hurried to the hospital to which Mr Manley had sent his wife. Before leaving, I phoned through and gave orders for an immediate X-ray. I told Mr Manley himself to meet me at the hospital in ten minutes.

In the meanwhile I picked up the house telephone and rang my secretary, who told me the whole of the mournful tale.

Edward Manley had apparently spent many precious seconds explaining to her how his wife had swallowed her top denture, a rare enough occurrence, but highly dangerous.

She had been eating a banana and that innocent fruit was the cause of the tragedy. There were exactly five teeth on the plate, Mr Manley had told the secretary, and at each end of the plate there were hooks.

The more I listened to the story the surer I was that the poor woman was very lucky to have survived at all. True to habit and fearful of an emergency operation, I 'phoned up the hospital again and got in touch with my house-surgeon. I told him to have the X-rays the moment I came in and to prepare the operating theatre. He was just about to elaborate some theory or other to me when I cut him short.

'Be over in ten minutes,' I said, 'and then you can spout your head off.'

In just over ten minutes a diminutive man, wringing his hands and sobbing, met me on the entrance stairs of the hospital. I recognized Mr Manley and shook him warmly by the hand, thereby probably restoring his circulation for him.

'I am the husband,' he said, as if he was a murderer. 'I gave her the banana.'

I could not help smiling at the poor little man's agony, but I knew it was no longer a laughing matter as far as the patient was concerned.

'It was a dreadful blow, a dreadful blow,' he kept on repeating. Then more earnestly he would moan, 'I've never hit her before in my life, but it was necessary, it was necessary.'

I agreed that it was and commended him on his promptitude. I looked at the little chap's muscles. He was very stockily built, and I was certain that he could deliver a pretty cruel blow at blow quarters.

I ran along the corridor with the harassed husband trotting behind me.

'You know,' he said, 'I've heard of cases where people swallow pins and needles and coins but never teeth – is it dangerous, doctor? Will my wife live?'

I made no answer but hurried into the private ward to see the patient.

I recognized her at first glance. She had been a patient of mine about two years previously. I think I had to make some slight correction to her nose, but I had lost touch with her and did not know of her being married. However, although I had forgotten her maiden name, I grinned broadly and said how do you do.

She appeared a little shy. I remembered now that I did not inquire whether her teeth were real or false when I did the last operation, because the plastic correction was done under a local anaesthetic. Had I used a general anaesthesia, I would have asked her as a matter of form. Anyway, she was so young-looking and so pink that no one would have thought she had false teeth. However, this wasn't a beauty competition.

The examination revealed that she had five front teeth missing, so that would mean a pretty large plate – together with hooks to keep it in place. Her throat was very badly scratched and there was some minor bleeding; but what was most amusing was that she was not complaining of any pain in her throat or her tummy, but kept on laying her hand on her back. Apparently the blow her husband had given her in saving, most probably, her life, hurt her far more than the severe scraping her throat got by the passing of the plate through it and the gullet.

The lady radiologist showed me the still-wet X-ray plates and my eyes nearly popped out when I beheld a dark object lying in the shallow, dark organ which was definitely the stomach. I could see that this object was very irregular and the two hooks looked magnified into pincers, so that the whole had the appearance of a small lobster.

It was obvious that the case was urgent. It seemed a miracle to me that the plate had managed to pass through the throat. Well, miracle or no miracle it had happened and what concerned me most was to get the plate out of the stomach.

For one thing was certain – that even if the gullet did let the unexpected object through, the pylorus – that is the narrow passage from the stomach into the intestine – certainly was not large enough for the plate to get through. There was no question of digesting five ivory teeth, and an ebonite plate with two metal hooks.

The pylorus, as a rule, is very muscular and yet at the same time delicate, and there was the certain danger of obstruction if the object was not taken out.

That would mean certain death. Secondly, there was an ever-present danger that the hooks would penetrate the soft linings of the stomach-walls and so cause peritonitis, again resulting in certain death.

Of course, I did not reason like this with the patient and her husband. I minimized the whole thing and assured them that, while an operation was imperative, if done in time it should not be dangerous.

To convince the husband I showed him the X-ray plates, which had the very opposite effect I had hoped for. He was terrified. I think he was most frightened by the word operation, although he did not have any other suggestions to make as to the alternative method of extracting the plate.

The patient herself was almost unable to give her consent. She merely referred me to Edward, and Edward seeing that there was no other way left, agreed and signed the consent.

The initial stages of the operation demanded what is called an upper abdominal laparotomy – an incision, that is – above the navel in the middle line of the body. When the stomach itself was exposed I was able to see that the organ was not empty but full of fluid – haemorrhage, probably caused by the hooks of the dental plate.

I selected the highest place on the anterior stomach wall on which to make the incision. I was careful to see that I was clear of all the big vessels and would do as little damage as possible.

Then I made my two-inch incision, and left it to my assistant to hold it open with two special hooks, called retractors. Then I managed to enter onto the stomach itself with long pincers and slowly and with great care I seized the plate and extracted it.

The contents of the stomach were sucked out with a special apparatus which was so designed as to prevent any leakage into the abdominal cavity. The incision was then closed with three layers of catgut, one row for each layer of the stomach wall. Half an hour later I was already out in the corridor assuring Edward Manley that his wife would be all right.

'The only inconvenience,' I said cheerfully, 'will be that your wife will walk about with a small scar in the middle of her tummy.'

But Edward Manley replied devoutly that he exonerated me completely and that if she lived, he would be eternally grateful to me, so, by way of a compliment, I commended him for his prompt action in beating his wife on the back.

'I would never have struck her but for my grandmother. She used to tell me that once her life had been saved by her husband thrashing her on the back – although I don't think it had anything to do with an artificial dental plate. He merely beat her because she had gone out unchaperoned, so I hardly can say that history has repeated itself ...'

It's amazing what sort of rot people talk when a great weight has been lifted off their minds.

'Do you know,' said Edward Manley, 'all this bother and

worry has given me a violent appetite? How about having dinner with me, Mr Sava?'

'No, Mr Manley,' I said. 'I have an appointment. But I'll take your lesson to heart and never offer a lady a banana.'

XII

The Unwanted Child

Much that happens to a surgeon is memorable. Yet only a few of the hundreds of faces he sees remain for ever engraved on his memory. Some for their beauty, some for their ugliness, some for the effervescent delight in life reflected in their eyes, and some for their absolute desolation. It is for this last reason that I shall always recall the face of Signora Mathilde Silvani on the first day I saw her. I shall also recall that first meeting because I was so entirely unprepared for its outcome. Particularly since I had been told by her doctor that it was not she who was to be my patient, but her newly-born baby.

Naturally, I expected her to be upset and worried. Indeed, what mother could fail to be when she discovers that her first baby is born with an unfortunate handicap? Even doctors are taken aback all over again each time a defective child is delivered. I, personally, have never been able to reconcile myself to these seemingly unjust failures of natures, let alone become detached or callous about them.

However, I have always found that the mother, sorely shocked and saddened at first, will soon be consoled when assured by her doctor that the deformity can be remedied. Nowadays this is especially true since the great advances in surgery, and many a deformity can be entirely corrected.

It was on a fine Monday morning that the doctor of a small clinic in the outskirts of Rome telephoned me. I was feeling particularly cheerful.

His downcast voice soon sobered me. 'Professor Sava, I have just delivered the first baby of my patient, Signora Silvani, and, unfortunately, the child has a harelip.'

'Poor woman,' I sympathized.

'Could you please come and see the baby as soon as you possibly can,' begged the anxious doctor.

I made arrangements to go to the clinic that evening after my consulting hours. The doctor sounded greatly concerned about his patient and it behoved me not to delay longer than could be helped. He, no doubt, had tried to console the mother and the fact that a plastic surgeon had been called in was ample evidence that the case was receiving every attention.

As far as I was concerned it was simply a case of another harelip no different from the numerous ones I had corrected in the past. To me a harelip is hardly a disaster that it used to be, since it can be corrected without too much danger of complications by plastic surgery. My meeting with Signora Salvini proved as disconcerting as it was unexpected.

The moment I set foot in the little clinic I sensed that something was amiss; something very much out of the ordinary must have taken place. The clinic, I knew, was a well-organized, peaceful home, but this time I felt that all was not well. The drawn, worried face of the doctor who met me in the entrance hall, the hustle and bustle of the usually calm sisters, the whisperings, by no means fitted into the normal atmosphere of the clinic.

'Oh, Professor Sava, I am so glad you have come,' exlaimed the doctor in a distressed tone.

'Why, has anything serious happened? Has the child been taken ill?'

'Oh no, the child is as well as could be expected. It's the mother. She is causing us all a great deal of worry. She is in such a dreadful state, *Professore*, we just dare not leave her alone for a minute for fear she does herself harm.'

'Because of her baby's harelip?'

'Well, it must be that. Her delivery was perfectly normal, and she seemed quite well in herself, too.'

I sympathized with the poor woman. No doubt it was a nasty shock; one somehow never expects deformities to happen to one's own child. 'Surely,' I said to the doctor, 'you have explained to her that it is not too difficult to correct a harelip nowadays?'

'Of course, *Professore*, I spent the whole day trying to make her see reason and that it was not such a catastrophe after all.' He shrugged his shoulders. 'I might just as well have been talking to myself. She does not even want to see her husband. She is in a frightful state and frankly I do not understand it. Perhaps you could help.'

'I will certainly try,' I said, following him to the patient's room.

As we ascended the stairs I reflected on what I had just been told. I sincerely hoped the emotional young doctor had exaggerated the patient's state of mind. If not, surely a third-floor room was hardly a wise choice for suicidal tendencies!

We entered softly. An immobile, mournful figure lay prostrate on the bed. Not the slightest reaction, not even a glance at our entry. She was obviously completely detached from her surroundings; her wide open eyes were fixed in a glazed stare on the ceiling. Now and again a deep sigh would escape her, then she would relapse once more into the kind of lethargy I had so frequently observed in advanced states of shock and depression.

This condition is particularly prevalent in young mothers, usually following a difficult confinement. Some women, as yet unaccustomed to motherhood, are often tormented by inexplicable dreads and doubts; nagging hidden fears beset them with such force that for a while they are almost on the verge of madness.

The doctor had certainly not exaggerated the state of Signora Silvani. Women in such a state entirely lack responsibility for their actions and can quite easily not only hurt themselves, but might even inflict injury on their baby. For in this disturbed state of mind they might well look upon the baby as the cause of all their misery.

The doctor cleared his throat and tried to assume a cheerful expression: '*Buona sera, Signora Silvani.*'

The eyes did not stir. There was no sign of recognition.

'I have brought Professor Sava to see you. The Professor is going to help your baby. Wouldn't you like to have a word with him?'

No reply came from the inert figure on the bed. Not a shadow of interest in her eyes.

'Doctor,' I said in a whisper, 'would you mind if I had a word with Signora Silvani alone?'

'Why, of course not!' he said with relief, glad to escape from this patient with whom he had spent so much time. 'I will wait for you downstairs.'

I turned to the nun still busying herself unnecessarily with some flowers in a vase. 'Sister, if you wouldn't mind leaving us now, I will call for you when I have finished.'

'Very well, *Signor Professore*,' she replied quietly, and followed the doctor out of the room.

Resolutely I walked to the window and opened it wide. The Roman night was overwhelmingly beautiful; the air was fragrant and pure, and a gentle breeze from the sea stirred the trees without.

I addressed the still figure: '*Signora*, you won't mind my opening the window, I hope. It is rather stuffy here. That's the trouble with hospital rooms – they all seem to have that peculiar odour of disinfectant and ether.' I inhaled noisily. 'Ah! that's grand! Do you by any chance live near here?' I drew up a chair to the bedside.

'Yes,' came the weak reply.

Hiding my surprise, I smiled at her encouragingly. 'It is lovely here, isn't it?'

'I live in Ostia,' she whispered.

'Ostia! That's a place I really love! Doesn't this air remind you of the sea?' If only I could keep the conversation flowing like this for a while, at least it would open up some possibility of closer communication.

'You know, *Signora*,' I remarked, 'whenever I manage to snatch a free evening – which does not happen often enough – I drive straight out to Ostia.'

I noticed for the first time a look of interest. Quickly I went on: 'I don't think there is a more pleasant way or a more relaxing way of spending an evening than to sit still and watch the setting sun gradually disappearing into the sea.'

Slowly, as if afraid, she turned her head to look full at me. For an instant I imagined I saw the faintest flicker of a smile.

Imagination or not, this indeed was encouraging.

'But you are not yourself a native of Ostia, are you, Signora Silvani?'

'No,' she said softly.

'Roman, perhaps?'

'Yes, from Travestevere.'

'Well, do you know, you are the first true Roman I have come across in all the five years that I have worked here. I was beginning to wonder if there were any genuine Romans left,' I laughed aloud, a foreign sound even to my own ears in that gloomy little room.

The soft, sorrowful smile around her mouth could not be mistaken. 'My husband was also born in Rome,' she told me in a voice that was a little more firm.

'Then you must have been childhood sweethearts?'

'Well,' she reflected, 'we did know each other as children, but we only became really friendly about a year before we were married.'

'And have you been married long?' I was quick to ask, for I felt we were broaching the subject that would reveal her secret.

'Yes – five years now.'

'And this is your first baby?' I knew the answer, but it was her reaction to the question, not the answer, that I wished to hear.

'Yes,' she managed to say, before bursting into heartbreaking sobs. 'God! I wish I were dead – oh, how I wish I were dead!'

For a moment I made no attempt to comfort her or even to stop her tears. It was the best cure for her at the moment; it would relieve her pent-up, soul-destroying emotions. For at least five minutes I sat there, watching the young mother unleashing her anguish and despair. I could scarcely remain untouched, but felt it wise to let her spend herself out.

She appeared an educated, intelligent woman who would hardly arrive at such a demented state solely on account of her baby's handicap, shock thought it must have been to her. I must discover, if I could, what was behind all this before I could help her.

When at last her sobs had changed to a pitiful whimper, I gently took her hand in mine.

'Please, *cara signora*, tell me a little more about yourself. I want to help you.'

I looked at her expectantly. Silence! I almost feared she might once more relapse into her former state of semi-coma, but was relieved to see her dabbing her eyes.

'What is there to tell you about myself? It couldn't interest you,' and again she repeated, 'Oh, I wish I were dead!'

'On the contrary, *signora*, it interests me very much, believe me. Remember, you are my first Roman patient, and there must be lots of things you can tell me. Please, I want to hear it.' Patting her hand, I added softly, 'Why are you so unhappy, *signora*?'

Her troubled eyes sought mine as if pleading for protection.

'Why am I so unhappy?' she repeated with a deep sigh. Again the tears started to flow. 'Oh, it's all my fault.'

'Do you mean about the baby?'

With tears streaming down her pallid cheeks, she told me with conviction that it was she, and she alone, who was to blame for the unfortunate baby's disfigurement; she should never have brought it into the world!

'Good heavens! What nonsense!' I said vehemently. 'As a doctor, I can tell you that no one, absolutely no one is to blame for such a mishap. Neither you nor your husband, nor anyone else. These things just happen and even we doctors do not know why.'

'That may be so in general. But with my baby it's different. I do happen to know why it happened.'

'You do?' I smiled. 'Then certainly you know more than I do!'

'Oh yes, I know all right,' she almost hissed, covering her face with her hands. 'It's all my fault,' she repeated. 'If only I hadn't done all those awful things ...'

'Now, *signora*, don't talk like that. You can't possibly blame yourself for something that no one can be blamed for.'

She buried her head in the pillows and amidst muffled cries the words came out. 'I didn't want him. That's why! I never wanted children at all!'

'Why not?' I persisted. 'You love your husband, don't you? Or did you think you couldn't afford to have children – you're not the only one, you know?'

'No, no,' she replied more calmly, her face turned to me once more. 'That wasn't it. We're well off. Only I was so selfish; I never stopped thinking about myself. All I wanted was a good time. I didn't want to be bothered with children and all the chores that go with them! That's why we didn't have any all those years.'

With a sad smile, I told her truthfully: 'that is not so unusual either, *signora*. Lots of women feel that way the first few years of their married life. But what made you change your mind?'

'That's just it! I didn't decide to have one. Roberto tricked me. He has always wanted children!'

'Well, I hardly think your husband is to be blamed for that. But you'll see all the fun there is to be had with a baby. When you are feeling better, you'll change your mind about everything.'

'Strangely enough, I don't really mind having the baby now; not after having been through the nine months' pregnancy and the confinement. But I was expecting a normal baby – a baby like anyone else's.'

I nodded in assent. 'It would certainly have been easier for you with a first child. But from what the doctor has told me, your baby is perfectly normal apart from this one affliction. And this, I promise you, I intend to remedy. And to you, its mother, your baby will be more beautiful than anyone else's – you'll see!'

'You don't know all,' she confessed with shame. 'When I realized I was pregnant I tried to prevent it. The amount of bitter pills and drugs I took! – anything I could lay my hands on. So you see, I really am to blame. It could have been a perfect baby but for me.'

So the truth was out! Her recrimination had not stemmed from superstition, but from ignorance. I felt it my duty to assuage her self-torture and save her from months of depressive illness.

For almost an hour I sat by her bedside, telling her of

various cases of harelip and other deformities children were frequently born with. Not only cases where prevention has been attempted, but in babies who were eagerly awaited by devoted mothers.

She listened intently, her eyes riveted on mine. Suddenly she asked: 'How can you be so certain the pills didn't do the damage? You yourself said you did not know the reasons for hare-lip – couldn't it have been the drugs I took?'

The fact that she not only listened, but was actually beginning to ask questions, convinced me that my endeavours were not in vain. The answer to her last question was of vital importance. Even if I had harboured some personal doubts about the possibility of injury being caused by drugs not medically prescribed, it would be fatal to reveal them here. I must not waver; must not show the slightest uncertainty, and must convince her positively.

'Oh no, *signora*,' I said firmly. 'In the case of hare-lip, it could not possibly be due to the drugs. Harelip is what we call a congenital deformity, and may happen to any baby. I have studied medicine for thirty years and can tell you that if the pills you took were really harmful they would have stopped your pregnancy. Your baby would never have been born.'

In her eyes was a startled and yet somewhat incredulous look.

'You must give me credit for knowing what I am talking about,' I continued.

The startled expression changed to one of profound relief. Her eyes betrayed a calmer, less disturbed frame of mind. We chatted for a while about things in general and I gradually turned the conversation to her married life, her husband and his work. She had become quite amenable and even seemed glad to be able to talk about herself at last.

I felt the time had now come to attempt my next hurdle. The doctor had told me earlier that she refused to see her husband and I was hoping to bring this young couple together again. This, I felt, could be achieved through their baby.

'*Signora*, where is your husband?' I asked. 'I would very much like to have a word with him.'

'Why?' She was instantly on the alert.

'Because, my dear, if you want me to operate on your baby I need not only your consent but your husband's permission also.'

'I see. Well, you can phone him. He will be at home now. But whatever happens, I don't want him to come here!'

'But you do want me to operate on the baby?'

'Of course, *Professore*,' she said firmly.

'Good! Then I will ask the sister to fetch him and we can examine him here!'

'No, no!' she cried in horror. 'Not here! I don't want to see him! For God's sake!'

'All right, all right!' I tried to calm her. 'But you will have to sign the form for permission to operate.'

'Yes, I'll sign.' She was still shaken at the thought of seeing the child.

I learnt when I left her that throughout all this time the husband had been sitting in the waiting-room. The doctor was with him. As I entered they both rose eagerly, their expectant eyes trying to read in my face what had happened in the room upstairs.

In a few words I assured them that Signora Silvani was far less distraught and had given me permission to operate on the child. Then I turned to Signor Silvani.

'You, too, will have to sign the form.'

'Certainly, *Signor Professore*!' he said sadly. 'Anything to help my child and poor Mathilde.'

'It will help, I can assure you. It is the only possible way of action,' I told him.

'Thank God!' he said fervently. 'Do you think I can go and see Mathilde?'

'I'm afraid not – not just yet, anyway.'

His face fell at this great disappointment.

'Your wife needs rest and quiet. Only the doctor should see her at present. You will see her soon enough,' I smiled. 'Just a little more patience.'

It was all I could do for the dejected man, but I felt sure that it would not be long before my efforts would show some more appreciable result.

'Now it is about time I saw my real patient,' I said to the

doctor. 'We must not forget him, must we?'

We left the father sitting miserably in his chair. What little hope I had been able to give him was recompensed with a grateful smile.

The baby was a fine, well-proportioned lad, weighing about seven pounds. Indeed, he would have been a lovely baby but for the ugly gap which split his upper lip, the upper jaw and the palate. This deformity could not have been more aptly named, resembling as it did in every detail the grotesque lip of a wild hare.

Poor Matilde, I thought, what an intense shock she must have received when her child was first placed into her arms! The child she had not wanted, so pitifully deformed. I placed my ear close to the chest of the baby. The heart beats were strong and healthy.

'I shall operate on him tomorrow,' I informed the doctor and asked him to assist.

'Tomorrow?' he repeated in surprise. 'You don't think it would be wiser to wait until he is a little older? He is only two days old now.'

'I agree it would be dangerous to carry out the whole operation in one so young,' I replied. 'I intend only to correct the lip itself so that the mother at least won't shrink from the sight of her child, and she may well begin to love it.'

The doctor reflected for a moment. 'And what about the cleft palate and the jaw, *Professore*?'

'That can wait, but not longer than a few months,' I emphasized. 'For if we wait too long, the child's speech will be impaired, and that will only add to our difficulties.'

'I see and understand, *Signor Professore*. I will see that everything is made ready for the operation.'

And thus baby Robertino was operated on at the ripe age of precisely three days. He was put to sleep by one of the ablest anaesthetists in Rome and the operation went smoothly.

I shortened one of the nostrils to correct the crooked nose – always an accompanying feature in harelip. The two halves of the upper lip were separated from the jaw; the edges were cut into straight lines, and then the two portions joined together.

The wound was left unbandaged. A small metal spring was

fixed to the baby's cheeks, arching over the mouth, thus leaving it free. If the baby cried, as inevitably it would, the wound would remain undisturbed and could not burst apart.

For ten days I visited my little patient and attended to him myself. Nothing must be left to chance. The smallest oversight might spoil the success of the operation. I even employed a special nurse to supervise the feeding of the baby, since this was a very complicated and exacting procedure.

At last came the long-awaited reunion of the parents. It was on the tenth day after the correction of their child's deformity. He was a truly lovely baby now, with only a red line to indicate where the harelip had previously been.

I looked at the speechless, elated father, standing in admiration, lost for words, his mouth agape.

'You have been admirably patient and brave all this time,' I said to him. 'But I think everything is going to be all right now. I would like you to come with me, and we will introduce your son to his mama.'

Three jubilant men walked into Signora Matilde Silvani's room – the young doctor, Signor Silvani and myself. Little Robertino made his entrance in his father's arms. We all had huge grins on our faces. A sister was standing by Matilde's bed attempting to calm the over-excited woman. Her face was averted in fear of what she might see, and our little procession was ignored.

'*Signora*,' I ventured. 'Now, don't tell me you don't want to see the *bello bambino*.'

'Darling,' cried the husband joyfully. 'Just look at him! He is perfectly beautiful – see for yourself!'

The nursing sister joined in the praises. 'He's a lovely baby.'

Slowly, warily, Matilde turned her head. Her eyes rested fleetingly on my face, then stopped short on the shiny little face of the bundle clutched so possessively in its father's arms. She sat up in bed, her muscles twitching, her eyes widening. Then an expression warmed her face: an expression of utter disbelief, of tender motherly pride, of joy! She opened her arms wide.

'Please, I want him!'

Her elated husband gladly handed the child to his mother. Greedily, almost, she embraced him, then gently pressed the fragile object to her bosom. Tears flowed down her cheeks, but this time they were tears of joy.

'*Dio mio*,' she whispered into the bundle. 'Please forgive me! Oh, forgive me!'

The words were meant also for her husband. Shyly she beckoned to him. As he approached closer, she grasped his hand.

'Sit by me, Roberto,' she whispered. 'Let us look at our beautiful baby together.'

XIII

Death Takes a Holiday

By all human standards of reckoning Sylvia Manning should have been dead! I shall forever fail to understand, therefore, how it came about that she was not. Unless at the time of her accident death had suddenly, on a lively impulse, decided on a little holiday. A short trip, maybe – a respite from its seasonless harvesting. Perhaps, then, just as its scythe had loomed over Sylvia Manning, death had downed tools and refused, for the moment, to harvest any more.

'Doctor Sava,' said the traffic-patrolman who had accompanied the ambulance. 'This time, I'm afraid, we're bringin' a corpse!'

As he became aware of my perplexed expression, he added hastily: 'I'm sorry, Doc! Sure, very sorry.'

'But why to us, man – why not straight to the mortuary?' I asked.

'They have to be certified as "stiffs" before a post-mortem can be made. Besides, we're – we're not all that sure that she, well, that she is all that dead! Are we Sam?' And he turned to his mate, the ambulance driver, for support.

'All right, Officer, don't worry!' I could not hide a faint smile at his ingenious choice of expression. 'Just bring her into the emergency room and I'll – I'll find out for you how dead she really is!'

I stood aside in the corridor while the two men carried the stretcher on which lay a lifeless bundle of humanity. At first glance the woman undoubtedly appeared to be dead. Lifeless, half-opened eyes, hair sticky with blood; one arm drooping limply over the side of the stretcher, as if it did not belong to her body. Not a sound or sign of breathing.

The officer, who still could not tear himself away from the gruesome sight, shook his head several times, in grim disbelief, then his boyish eyes caught mine.

'Lord Almighty!' I exclaimed. 'It does look as if you were right! Just how in heaven's name did this happen?'

He swallowed hard. 'Aw – y'know these looney dames ...' His effort at unconcerned cynicism was ill-suited to the shocked, almost frightened expression in his eyes. 'Drivin' at a hundred per hour; they're jus' beggin for trouble! Bust tyre and off she goes over the rails!'

'It can bring terrible tragedy, careless driving!' I said, bending over the motionless figure. 'You know, it frightens me too – every time I see a thing like this.'

'I'd better leave you to it, then, doctor.'

'Yes, officer. You go into the waiting-room and have a cup of coffee. I'll let you know my findings as soon as I can.'

I had now been at this hospital for three weeks and never yet had a day passed without my being faced with some form of road accident. The effect on me was such that, for the first time in my entire driving career, I really began to fear the roads!

The most apt words could never have convinced me half so poignantly or half so forcefully of the folly – or rather the crime – of reckless driving. Confronted daily with its victims, even if I did not immediately throw my car keys out of the window, at least I was learning a lesson I would remember with a nauseating, bitter taste for the rest of my days!

I resolved never again to take risks or to drive negligently, as admittedly I had done on more than one occasion. A tragic aspect of all this is the fact that somehow one never connects oneself, even in the slightest, with such savage disasters – they happen only to others! It is only when those others are lying before you, lifeless and disfigured beyond all recognition, that the stark possibility suddenly becomes a reality: 'This could be you!' It is only then that it is brought home to you how brazenly you brush against death yourself each day of your life!

Very often now, when my wife or son chanced to be home

late and had taken the car, I grew uncomfortably hot under the collar. I had made them promise me faithfully never to exceed the American fifty-five miles speed limit and always, in all circumstances, to keep a clear two cars' distance from the other automobiles. In return, I gave them the same promise. Not knowing, of course, that only two years later I would be a victim to a car accident and nearly lose my own life!

Today's disaster, however, was the ugliest I had so far had to witness! As I followed the sorry little procession into the emergency room, I was joined by Mike Schultz, the owner of the hospital and his senior resident house-man, Gregory Wise.

'Well, Dr Sava,' said Dr Wise, turning to me. 'I don't think you'll be wanting my help with this poor creature!'

'It does look that way, Wise, but – you never can tell! Just hang on another minute, will you? Let's carry out the examination first!'

I borrowed Dr Schultz's stethoscope and asked the nurse to unbutton the woman's blouse. With the stethoscope placed over her chest and my ear glued to the instrument, I listened, without much hope, for a few seconds.

As I handed the stethoscope to Mike, the only remark I passed was: 'Here, Mike, listen, will you?' I deliberately withheld from him the reason for wanting his opinion. For it had seemed to me that I could discern the faintest of heartbeats!

I thought this impression so illogical at the time that I put it down to my vivid imagination – yet, without influencing Mike, I none the less wanted his verdict. Intently I watched for any change of expression on Mike's face. Was I right – was there a look of alertness – was he listening a second time with renewed interest? Sure enough, he straightened once, then instantly bent over the woman again, to resume his listening. Again he straightened, and spoke at last:

'You heard it too, didn't you, George?'

'Yes, I did, but it seemed such an impossibility – I just couldn't trust my own ears. At any rate, I wanted you to confirm or deny it!'

Even now, like myself, Mike was unable to credit the sounds of breathing from a woman who, in ever other way, had nothing in common with a living human being. He put the stethoscope into Dr Wise's hand. 'See if you can hear it too, Greg!'

More silence, suspense, baited breath as Wise bent over her! Yet quicker than either of us had done, he confirmed our conjecture with a decisive nod. 'You aren't imagining things – I can definitely hear heartbeats and breathing!'

So Sylvia Manning really was not yet 'quite dead'! Unwittingly, the patrol officer had come very near the truth, when he had remarked that he wasn't 'really sure that she's all that dead!'

More than likely the shock of the severe internal injuries was responsible for her condition. It was quite clear to all of us present, that although she was not yet dead, the end could not be far off. Unless – unless something very drastic could be done immediately.

We required no discussion or further consultation to agree on our next step. We all knew that if it were humanly possible, we intended to discover this drastic way which would restore Sylvia Manning to the world of the living, instead of oscillating somewhere between the two worlds, as she was at present.

The moments of doubt and indecision were gone and their place was taken by a rush of orders and bustling activity. An oxygen cylinder was rushed in and its mouth-piece connected to the patient. Heart stimulants were directly injected into her veins.

Again those interminable, anxious moments of waiting! Then a very, very timid touch of colour actually began to creep into her hitherto chalk-white cheeks, Now her chest started to heave; at first with a shallow, but soon with a deeper and more regular rhythm.

As softly and painstakingly as I knew how, I went over her body with my fingers. The list of her injuries – discovered and suspected – began to sound like a text book.

'Multiple lacerations of face, arms and body,' I dictated to Dr Wise. 'Comminuted fractures of left arm, wrist and possible fracture of left leg and left ankle,' I continued. 'Probably severe internal injuries, with internal bleeding.'

Turning towards my colleagues for a moment, I said urgently:

'With this last, as you no doubt realise, we must deal instantly – if we are to have any hope of saving this woman!'

'That would be nothing short of a miracle,' muttered Greg Wise to himself.

'It would indeed! But all the same, that's just what we've got to try to bring about – we must try to save this poor woman!'

'Of course, Dr Sava, but it looks unbelievably hopeless right now!'

'What exactly d'you think her internal injuries are?' Mike Schultz inquired of me, while he felt her abdomen with that wonderfully gentle touch of his.

'Most likely rupture of the spleen,' I hazarded. 'It appears that her injuries are chiefly concentrated on the left side of her body. But I wouldn't by any means exclude injuries to the liver and stomach, especially if the poor woman had a substantial meal before her accident!'

Schultz heard me to the end without saying anything further. This was a case for surgery and with his usual courtesy he waited for me to offer my surgical suggestions. As usual, also, he had not long to wait.

'Come on, Mike – let's get her to the operating theatre!' I told him forcefully. 'You will give the anaesthetic, won't you? There just isn't time to wait for the anaesthetist.'

'Why, of course, George, I'll be glad to! Let's get weaving then!' I felt that Mike had expected me to react in exactly this way and the knowledge strengthened my determination.

Fortunately the technician had just finished verifying the patient's blood group and I could order several pints of blood. I asked Dr Wise to begin the blood transfusion immediately. At the most, half an hour had elapsed between the time Sylvia Manning had arrived at the hospital and the time when she lay on the operating table before us. Two pints of blood flowed simultaneously into her right arm and leg. And thus began another of the innumerable tussles between the surgeon's knife and death!

Being uncertain of the exact nature of the internal injuries, I decided to open the abdomen with a large, mid-line incision;

in this way I would gain access to all the abdominal organs. If, until now, I had harboured some small hope of saving this woman's life, this hope was now to fail me as I saw the severe havoc contained within the abdomen.

All that confronted us was a deep crimson sea of blood; nothing was distinguishable but this flood of crimson liquid. Very dark blood it was, with ominous, dreaded yellow streaks – bile! To begin with, therefore, we could reckon with damaged liver and gall-bladder.

'What next?' I asked myself, as I began carefully to suck the blood away with the electric aspirator. Gradually, with painful slowness, the abdominal cavity was cleared, and one by one the abdominal organs became visible.

On the left-hand side, under the lower ribs, we discovered, instead of the small, pink organ the spleen should have been, a mass of disintegrated tissue! A rupture of the spleen – more of an explosion than a rupture, for that matter!

At that moment, I could ill afford to spend more time on detailed inspection of intestines, stomach and kidneys. First and foremost, the spleen and liver had to be dealt with. Moreover, this had to be done with great speed if the bleeding was to be controlled. Luckily, in only a few minutes, we located the stump of the spleen, origin of most of the bleeding. Veins and arteries were ligated and pieces of the spleen removed. This put an end to the bleeding from one source at least; now came the liver!

The gall-bladder, torn beyond repair, had to be removed. The liver was cut in three places as if by a sharp knife. These cuts we cleansed and gently sutured. This procedure succeeded in stifling the bleeding from the second source. 'Let it be the last,' I prayed silently.

Now I could resume inspection of the remaining organs. Here, at last, we were to meet with considerably more encouragement. For stomach and intestines appeared quite unimpaired. The left kidney, though bruised, did not reveal irreparable damage.

'Thank God for that!' This time I spoke aloud. 'Let's close up the abdomen!' I said to Greg Wise, who was assisting me. 'How are you doing?' I suddenly remembered to ask Mike.

Until then, I had been so engrossed in my work that even to enquire how he was faring with his anaesthetic had literally slipped my mind!

'Not too bad – not too bad at all, surprisingly enough, George,' Mike told me. 'She's holding her own!'

Another fifteen minutes and the first part of Sylvia's resurrection was concluded. It had, in all, taken the best part of two hours. 'Well, Greg, so far so good. Perhaps the age of miracles is not yet past! Hm?'

'For the life of me, I wouldn't have believed it possible that she should still be alive!' He paused and looked me straight in the eye. 'But – even now – do you really believe she'll pull through?'

I met his glance with equal seriousness as I replied: 'I don't know, Greg; how can I tell? We can only do our job, the rest is in God's hands.'

Indeed, it could only have been God's Will, which in the end seemed almost to drag Sylvia Manning back to life and engineered her amazing survival! In cases such as these, where life hangs so precariously in the balance, I always like to imagine that someone very close to the sufferer has prayed with reverence, devotion and humility. To me it seems that only such anguished tears, such love and faith, can truly stir the heart of God, to bring about the real victory.

The patrol-officer, who had sat in the waiting-room all this time, was by now drinking his umpteenth cup of black coffee and puffing great clouds of smoke from his never-ending supply of 'Camels'. With him in the room, when I entered, were several other people. Just then, however, I was far too preoccupied to take much notice of them. 'Would you please come outside for a moment,' I addressed the officer.

He rose instantly, obviously relieved that I had not completely forgotten him; had not the nurse reminded me, in all truth I would have done just that! Anyway, I now took him by the arm and led him along the corridor into the doctors' room.

'If you've got your book ready, I can give you some more particulars of Sylvia Manning!'

This young patrol-officer – a profession which in itself, so I had always imagined, requires a certain amount of courage, or callousness, call it what you will – smiled at me with the gentle, sad smile of a school-master. His wide blue eyes were the eyes of a kind-hearted, sensitive human being: I could not help wondering what had made him choose this far from gentle profession of his.

'I'm ready, Doc, I've been ready for hours,' he subtly rebuked me.

'I'm sorry you've had to wait so long, but I couldn't give you all the information until now. She's alive, you know,' I added as an afterthought, suddenly recollecting that this young man thought he would be given details of the death of Sylvia Manning.

Maybe I should have prepared him, for he was quite stunned, his eyes fairly popping out of his head.

'Alive!' he exclaimed. 'Really alive! Jeez, Doc, if that ain't the most – the most ...'

'Amazing, eh?' I came to the confounded lad's rescue.

'Amazin' – you said it!' Then a thought struck him. 'Doctor, could you please come and tell her hubby and kids the wonnerful news yourself?'

I thought this over for a while. 'Well, son, I'm not so sure, yet, that it is such wonderful news!'

'Gee, Doc!' He nearly jumped at me in his childish enthusiasm. 'It is swell – it's just the greatest news! Cain't you see, they think their Maw is dead, anyway! Now, now there's hope!'

Here was a so-called 'hard-boiled' officer with a genuine affection for people; I don't think, at this point, that I would have been astonished if he had wiped away a tear or two. I, for one, was glad that there were men of sentiment to be found even in the profession where feelings are generally pooh-poohed.

'Of course! You're right, young man! I'll do it straight away!'

When a heart-broken, ashen-faced husband and three terrified, bewildered children stood before me, I found myself making a doubly strong resolve to try to save Sylvia Manning. If humanly possible, this woman must be spared – it would wipe away the look of anguish on the faces before me.

Not till much later was I to learn exactly how Sylvia Manning had managed to become the battered wreck she was. She had completely lost control of the car after a tyre had burst and everything had just gone berserk.

Three times the car had somersaulted, to end up with a terrible crash by the trunk of a tree. The car itself had to be scrapped for junk – Sylvia Manning lived! Such are the inscrutable whims of fate.

Not that we did not have more than our share in her recovery!

Sylvia stayed at our hospital for three months. Once her internal injuries had been dealt with, X-rays helped to detect all the fractures in her body. We soon discovered she had five fractured ribs – but, incredible as it may sound, the lung itself had remained intact!

In addition, of course, came the fractures we already knew of: in arms, legs, hands and feet. Not a little labour was there for us, if Sylvia was one day to resume a normal, active life as a wife and mother.

The clearer our path became, the happier became our work. Some of the fractures were fixed with metal plates; the arm was put into a plaster of Paris cast and the leg suspended over the end of an extension apparatus.

So we, as well as Sylvia Manning herself, fought desperately for her life during the following two months. Sometimes she may have complained – and certainly she had much to complain of; yet this was an unmistakable sign of improvement and recovery and we were glad to see it!

Most of the time, however, Sylvia's relationship with all of us was one of deep gratitude and intelligent, almost touching endurance. She bore all her tribulations stoically, and undoubtedly the pain and discomfort must at times have been unbearable.

At long last, Sylvia's ordeal was at an end. Everything was mending, her youth contributing immensely to her final recovery. For Sylvia Manning was only thirty-five years old and had, until the day of her accident, been an exceptionally healthy, happy wife and mother.

All the more reason to rejoice at her being spared!

How tragic, how senseless and futile it would have been, had a woman so much needed and loved been snatched from life at one plundering swoop!

Obviously God in His great mercy and understanding, had heard the anguished husband's prayers and the innocent children's love for their mother.

We were only the tools He chose for saving the life of Sylvia Manning.

XIV

The Love Birds

The day I met the first of two of the most lovable characters in my case-book was memorable not solely for the lady's appearance on my medical horizon. For that day was also to mark a vital change in my life as a California surgeon.

It was the beginning of September. The morning was one such as only California could conjure up – California at its superb best! The sun was warm, but no longer so hot that it rendered work an unpleasant burden. The clear blue sky was visible for endless miles; for on this day it was completely devoid of the infamous Californian smog.

To tell the truth, throughout my stay in California, I never could quite make out what all the fuss was about when people complained of 'that dam' awful smog!' Newspapers were always full of disparaging remarks about it; radio and television announcers cursed it. The only reason, as far as I could see, which might have caused this public outcry was a slight haze in the air obscuring the brightness of the sun and causing one's eyes to smart very slightly. I swear that was all! But then, few Californians have experienced autumn or winter in London or the Midlands – so how could they possibly know the true meaning of mist and fog?

Yet on this particular day there was not a trace of smog. Already on the point of leaving for the hospital, I could not refrain from standing for a while at the open French windows. Spellbound, I gazed into space, enveloped by the comforting warmth and scent of the flowers from the garden. There was really no need to rush, for there had been little activity at the hospital of late. No doubt the sudden slump in work was caused by the rumours that had been circulating for the past few weeks. Everyone seemed to have heard about the impending changes in both the hospitals's administration and its medical organization.

For my part, however, I was not unduly troubled by this respite. After all, a little leisure after constant hard work was hardly unwelcome. I had still barely recovered from that 'taste of hell' the terrible car accident had brought me, and considered this unexpected rest as almost a gift of the gods.

Nevertheless, I felt it my duty to leave home at my usual hour of eight. This was a hospital – one never could tell from one minute to the next what might crop up! Just as I was about to close the front door behind me, the telephone began to ring. A call at this early hour did not surprise me since it had frequently occurred in the past. The reception clerk at the hospital had orders to notify me the moment an emergency case was brought in.

The surprise, therefore, was not the actual phone call, but the voice greeting me from the other end of the line. For I soon recognized it as that of Mike Schultz himself.

'Not another misfortune like that last one, surely?' I could not help worrying fleetingly. 'But why would Mike phone me at this time of the morning?'

His first words, however, were sufficient to put me at my ease and allay all fears of an unwelcome spurt of work. For in his usual friendly tone Mike said:

'What are you supposed to be doing at the hospital this morning?'

'Oh, nothing much; nothing special, anyway!' And I told him, 'One appendix and one hernia – I think that's the lot!'

'Perfect!' he exclaimed. 'I'm sure Greg Wise can see to them, don't you agree?'

'Of course he can, but why shouldn't I do them?'

'Because, my dear George, I have taken the liberty of officially giving the two of us the morning off!'

'Mm, that sounds like good news! Ahem – what's the catch?'

Mike began laughing at my last question, though I failed to see its particular merits as a joke. Amidst guffaws, he managed to say at last:

'What's the catch, he says! You've just about hit the nail on the head – you see, pal, you and I are about to go on a little fishing trip!'

Just for a moment, I was so astonished that I stood dumbfounded with the receiver in my hand.

Mike must have interpreted my silence as reluctance, for in a disappointed voice he now inquired, 'I thought you loved fishing, George, don't you?'

Now I suddenly awoke to the joke I had earlier made so unintentionally. Roaring heartily, I told Mike: 'Now I see the joke! Do I love fishing – you bet I do! It was just such a surprise that it knocked the wind out of me!'

'Swell! Then you get on the phone to Greg straight away and ask him to take over those two operations. I'll pick you up in about twenty minutes, OK?'

'Very much OK, Mike, thanks. I'll be ready!'

As it happened, the twenty minutes only just sufficed. The various instructions I had to give to Dr Wise took up almost fifteen of them, so that I had only five minutes left in which to make a quick change into something suitable for the fishing expedition ahead.

As good as his word, Mike's car roared up to the gate, punctual to the minute. I took my seat beside him, banged the door with gusto and off we sped to Long Beach, where Mike kept his motor-boat anchored. And so it came about that for one morning I became a Californian fisherman!

Unfortunately I am not much more than a novice where fishing is concerned. Much as I relish the peaceful, soothing effect it has upon me, I have never found the time to take it up seriously. Thus the first half-hour in Mike's boat had to be devoted to his teaching me the ABC of the proper use of the fishing-rod.

I wonder if there is a more enchanting way of whiling away a morning than by gently floating across the Pacific Ocean, a couple of miles out from the shore – and hundreds of miles away from the hectic everyday world! That day the Pacific Ocean really lived up to its name, not a breeze stirred, not a wave rippled. Endless calm, endless beauty! Time was unimportant here; twentieth century or fifteenth – there was nothing except the boat itself to betray what era we had strayed from.

It was almost unreal in its vast perfection. The sea, silken smooth, had the crystal clarity of a giant looking-glass used solely for reflecting the golden splendour of the sun and the azure innocence of the sky. It made an unforgettable moment, stirring just because of its unsurpassed tranquillity. One is inclined to forget in the mad hubbub of modern life what peace there is still to be found in the gentle arms of nature!

Mike and I lounged on deck and cast our hooks lazily, with the bait trailing carelessly behind. Four hours of quiet happiness.

And what of the catch? In this part of the Pacific Ocean it is something that surely even the best, most expert of fishermen can only dream about! Short of experiencing it for oneself, it is hard to credit! After that fairy-tale day, I shall never again dare to doubt the tales of fabulous catches fishermen will sometimes astound you with – if, that is, these tales refer to the Pacific Ocean!

In those four hours, and with all my lack of experience, I was to hook no less than sixteen three-and four-pounder fish in all! The whole procedure was simply too good to be true; it was for all the world as if the fish were vying with each other for the honour of taking a nibble at the line of the hospital's chief surgeon. Not that they spurned the line of the hospital's owner by any means. In fact, we were forced to stop by mid-day or the boat might well have capsized with its enormous, fishy load. There were literally piles of different kinds of exotic fish in every corner – a morning's catch to be proud of for two medical fishermen.

With the assistance of the Mexican deck-hand we loaded our booty, stacked in two huge boxes, into the rear of the car. All the way home we kept a jealous guard on our prized treasure, thrilled as two schoolboys.

By then Mike had already divulged to me the second surprise he had planned. Of course, I knew that the hospital was about to change hands. What I did not know, however, was that Mike had arranged a meeting between the new owners and myself over lunch that same day.

What a frantic rush the moment I reached home, to clothe myself in attire more seemly and appropriate to the sober atmosphere of a fashionable Los Angeles restaurant. I could hardly risk the embarrassment of seeing the raised eyebrows at the spectacular entrance of a portly foreign surgeon – in blue fish-smelling jeans!

An hour later Mike's car drew up outside my house once more. This time we were to speed inland on our way to Los Angeles. To my poor house-keeper fell the rather unattractive smelly task of sorting out my fishy spoils and sorting them for the deep freeze.

The lunch turned out to be a relaxed informal gathering. There were three people involved in the take-over of the hospital. Over fried steak of sword-fish, with the introductions long since behind us, I was told that no special changes were contemplated in medical staff.

'Particularly not as far as you are concerned,' one of the three gentlemen told me, beaming.

'Why, thank you, gentlemen – I appreciate that,' I smiled in return. 'I only hope I won't disappoint you in any way.'

'On the contrary,' they insisted in unison. 'Mike just never stops singing your praises,' the first gentleman informed me. 'The only thing that worries us is that you yourself may not be so happy at the change.'

'Well, to be quite frank, I can't say I'm elated at the prospect of having to lose old Mike here – he's not the worst of bosses, you know!'

For a moment I looked over at Mike and felt a sinking, unpleasant sensation in the pit of my stomach.

'Still,' I added hastily, 'I shan't let that interfere with my work!'

'Fine. Can we take that as settled, then, Dr Sava?'

'You'll stay on, then?' This last question from the third and most determined of the trio.

'Yes, I think so – but –' I hesitated. 'I really would appreciate it if you could give me a week in which to discuss things with my family – you see, I do have rather a demanding one!' I smiled apologetically.

'Why, sure, Dr Sava, you just take your time, take all the time you need! Anyway, we won't be taking over for another month yet.'

Alone in the car with Mike, I asked: 'What do you think – could I make a go of it with them, could we work in harmony?'

'Yes, George,' he said slowly, 'I do believe you could. They may take some getting used to, especially since there are three of them – but I believe it would work out OK.'

'That's the feeling I have, too,' I admitted.

When I finally arrived at the hospital, it was past four. My day's work, though not even begun yet, was almost over. There was just time enough to make my rounds and plan the operating list for the next day.

While I was seated at the desk in my office, busy with the itinerary, the nurse on duty came to inform me that a lady was waiting to see me. 'All right, nurse, send her in, please!' I certainly could not complain of overwork that day!

A nice, unassuming little woman soon took her seat opposite me. She was about forty years old and seemed slightly nervous at first, hastening to apologize for not having made an appointment beforehand.

'I just came on the off-chance, doctor – on an impulse, like! You see, if I made an appointment I might not have the courage to keep it the next day,' she tried to explain, 'I do hope you don't mind me bursting in on you like this!'

'Now don't you worry about it – we doctors expect people to come and see us when they feel they need us – that's what we're here for, after all.'

A relieved smile appeared on the lady's face. 'I'm Mrs Sheena McCullough,' she now introduced herself. 'I do so hope you'll be able to help me, Doctor!'

'So do I, Mrs McCullough! Now then, how about telling me what is troubling you?'

'There's nothing really wrong with me – I can't say I'm sick in the ordinary way – but I've been told I need an operation!'

This last piece of intelligence took me somewhat by surprise; for the lady facing me looked far from ill, with her clear eyes and glowing skin. 'Who told you that you need an operation? You look remarkably fit to me, I must say!'

'Well, doctor, a gynaecologist examined me some years back and it was he who told me that if I wanted any more children I'd have to have this operation.'

'Oh, I see. How many years ago was that?'

'I'd say four years now, Doctor.'

'And – and you waited all this time, Mrs McCullough?'

'Yes, I'm afraid so, and I've got to admit I was rather scared of the operation at the time!'

Here she faltered and I could not help noticing the deep blush which was spreading over her face.

'Anyway,' she resumed, 'there wasn't much sense in my having anything done till now. I – I'm not married yet!'

She was Mrs MacCullough; four years ago she had asked to be examined by a gynaecologist, presumably because she wanted children – and she was not even married! Curiouser and more curiouser!

'You're a widow, Mrs McCullough?' I suggested helpfully.

'No, doctor, I'm divorced. But – again that schoolgirl blush – 'I shan't be single much longer now!' By her expression I could see that she loved her prospective husband a good deal, whoever the mysterious Romeo might be.

'And this time I'll make sure that he won't want to divorce me again! That's really why I'm here – to have the operation as soon as possible!'

As Mrs McCullough unfolded her story further, it was to grow more and more interesting. She had apparently been married for ten years and had given birth to one child – a daughter. Not wishing to have any more children, she had resorted to the use of various kinds of contraceptives – all without the knowledge of her husband. When he found out he was exceedingly angry, and this, according to Mrs McCullough, had caused the collapse of her marriage.

As if to add insult to injury, the poor woman had then been informed by a gynaecologist that her only hope of having any more children lay in an operation. Thus the McCulloughs had divorced four years ago.

By far the most curious part of all this, however, was revealed when I asked who her new spouse was to be.

'Why, my first husband – who else, doctor?' she replied

with all the innocence of a child, as if it were the only proper step to take for a divorced woman. 'I never stopped caring for him, never!' she impressed upon me. 'And I don't think he's ever looked at another woman either. Oh, he's a fine man!'

'What luck,' she continued – 'I'm quite sure it was God's doing – that we met again by chance in a cinema of all places! Would you believe it, doctor?'

I shook my head.

'After that, lonely as we both were, we soon realized what stubborn, silly fools we'd been – you know what I mean, don't you?' She giggled.

Again I could only nod.

I now examined Sheena McCullough carefully and found my verdict to be exactly the same as that of the gynaecologist. I realized that both of the uterine tubes were blocked. I therefore made arrangements for Mrs McCullough to have her operation the following week; for Sheena of the girlish blushes was most eager to have it performed as quickly as possible. 'You must promise me,' were her parting words. 'not to tell my husband that I'm going to have this operation!'

'Of course not, Mrs McCullough, if that's what you wish,' I promised.

Two days later I was to receive yet another visit from a McCullough. Again no appointment had been fixed, so this second McCullough had also apparently come on the 'off-chance'. This time it was one Ian McCullough who seated himself in the same chair occupied only a short while previously by my first McCullough.

Ian McCullough was a man of about forty-five, of medium height and with sandy-coloured hair. He looked the part of a true McCullough, even to the beak-like curve of his nose. From the moment we had shaken hands Ian McCullough showed himself to be a friendly, likable sort of fellow. And from the very first words he uttered there was no mistaking his origin, name and nose apart, even. For he had retained a very marked Scottish intonation and his expressions and mannerisms were very much more Gaelic than American.

'How are ye, doctor?' he had wanted to know as soon as he had set foot in my office. 'I do hope ye'll not mind my coming to see ye like this, with nae even an appointment.'

I assured him that he was welcome.

'What can I do for you, Mr McCullough?' I asked, quite convinced that this McCullough also was about to spring some surprise on me. Like his female namesake, he looked the picture of health.

'Were you recommended to come here by anyone?'

'Well, not exactly, Dr Sava,' he admitted. 'Though I've heard no end about ye from ma friends. Then when I looked ye up in the Medical Register and saw ye'd studied in guid old Glasgy – och well, I knew for certain that ye were the man for me!' And with a proud smile, he added: 'Ye canna beat Scottish surgery, eh?'

I, too, had to smile; the man's pride in his native land was touching. 'There's something in what you say, Mr McCullough – I am rather proud of having taken my fellowship in Glasgow, I must admit!'

'Now then, as one Scot to another,' I ventured, with what I knew to be a rather sorry imitation of the real Scottish accent, 'how can I help you?'

Ian McCullough appeared to be searching for words. 'It's like this, Dr Sava – ahem – I – I'm about to wed; och – ye know!' He smiled coyly. 'And it's ma old lass I'm being wed to!'

The dear man was very embarrassed now. I, on the other hand, had solved my puzzle. There could be no doubt that here we had Sheena McCullough's 'Darby' in the flesh! The only thing still remaining to be solved was the actual cause for his visit to me. For an unpleasant moment I had fears that he might somehow have found out about Sheena's impending operation and already had visions of myself as meddling between the two lovers. However, nice man that he was, he did not keep me too long in suspense.

I learned that Ian was quite convinced that the blame for the break-up of their marriage was his alone. For himself, he had never ceased adoring his lass. The strange thing was that he did not even find it of sufficient importance to mention the trouble they were supposed to have had over Sheena's refusal to give birth to any more children. To her it had seemed to be the crux of the matter; to Ian, however, it did not even warrant mentioning.

Mr McCullough had other ideas as to what had actually ruined his marriage. For his part, he put it all down to his ungainly looks.

'My wife's a bonny lass, doctor; just wait till ye see her – I'm sure ye'll agree!'

I now became George Sava the actor, feigning utter ignorance of his wife's appearance, 'bonny' or otherwise, and looking as blank as a veritable simpleton.

'I'm perfectly sure she could nae abide the sight of ma nose and ears any longer – that's why she left me, Doctor!' Sorrowfully, he pointed to the offending features.

His nose I had noticed already; undoubtedly it was of quite some size, not to mention the very steep curve it sported. As I scrutinized him more closely, I had also to admit that his ears could well be described by the unkind as 'donkey's ears', so large and protruding they were! True enough, Ian McCullough could not boast of film-star looks, yet I knew better than to believe that his ungainly nose and ears were the culprits in the upheaval of the McCullough home.

Besides, he was a most likable man, with his unaffected, natural ways. I agreed, nevertheless, to change his nose and ears for him, if only to relieve him of his firm belief that they had been the cause of his marital failure.

'I'm more than grateful, doctor – ye've been very helpful and understanding. That's what Scottish training does for ye, eh?' he said with a twinkle in his eye. 'But seriously, Dr Sava, do ye think that Sheena and I will be all right this time?' Happy anticipation lit up his whole face.

'I certainly hope you will, Mr McCullough!'

Just as he was about to walk out of the door, he suddenly turned to say: 'Ye will – ye must promise me, Dr Sava – not to tell me wife that I'm goin' to have this operation.'

Birds of a feather! I could have laughed out loud – word for word, he repeated his wife's parting phrase! His request, however, seemed almost ludicrous to me. Surely not only his wife, but everyone who knew him at all, would be bound to remark on his changed appearance – how then could he hope to keep it a secret from his wife of all people? Perhaps his motive was to spring a surprise on her, once his looks were improved. Be that as it may, he had expressed his wish and I, for one, would respect it.

Like his Sheena, he too had been most eager for an immediate operation. I now had to make hasty mental calculations – whatever happened, their times at the hospital could not be allowed to coincide!

I was successful with my correction on Ian McCullough's face. I had operated on Ian first so that the bruises would be gone by the time he 'wed his old lass'. His nose and ears were now positively handsome – an asset to his face! No sensible lass would take objection to this good-looking Scotsman, especially when he already possessed such a delightful disposition.

How successful Sheena McCullough's operation was, would take time to tell. But I was to find myself a guest at their remarriage. My position at this feast was a somewhat delicate and awkward one. I had pretended to each that I had never so much as set eyes on the other, and was merely a friend of one of them – of which one, I pride myself that I managed to keep rather vague.

*

Months had passed since the day I flew from Samoa to San Francisco and accepted the position of chief-surgeon at the Prince's Gate hospital – months that brought with them a great many changes.

It began with the letter I received full of congratulations for the successful operations on Daphne. Her family physician and friend wrote to me that he had spoken of me to people at various hospitals where he worked. He promised me that any one of them would be pleased to have me on their staff.

It all added up to a marvellous end to my stay in the USA. Or so I imagined. But when did things ever work out for me as imagined?

My stay in Australia ended and my thoughts strayed and came to a halt when they reached California. I still had the letter of congratulations. In it the surgeon gave the names of three hospitals which were keen to have my services.

I thought it might be interesting to see if they were still interested. From Samoa I wrote a short letter to the superintendent of the first hospital mentioned in the letter. It was a new, smallish establishment in the Northern part of California. To my delight, I received a reply by return of post. After stating details of the work done at the hospital, and telling me that he had heard of my success with the automobile accident cases, the man concluded with a plea:

'Please come as soon as convenient!' The salary offered plus portion of fees of private patients requiring plastic surgery was so inviting that I could not resist. To borrow a phrase from the Godfather – 'They made me an offer I could not refuse.'

And so I found myself working at the Prince's Gate hospital owned by Dr Michael Schuhz. I liked the man the moment we met.

'I am Michael Schultz,' he said smiling, 'Mike to my friends.' We shook hands. 'Welcome to California,' he beamed with enthusiasm.

'Glad to be here,' I said. 'It seems that I am destined to live and work in California.'

'It is to our great advantage, and a pleasure to have you with us.'

'I'm honoured, Dr Schultz.'

'The honour is ours, Dr Sava.'

And so my work began. It consisted of five mornings of surgery; on call every second weekend for emergencies and two afternoons for consultations and examination of outpatients at the clinic. The salary was quite generous. The offer was almost identical to the one I had had at the Santa Clara Hospital down south, where the FBI man was my first patient.

I did enjoy my work at the new hospital, but more I enjoyed the friendship Dr Mike Schultz gave me wholeheartedly. But now Mike was leaving and new owners were taking over.

What was I to do? On this, sixteenth of September, I gazed through the window of my bedroom. No rain to sneer at me, no dismal, leaden sky! Instead, there was the free azure horizon and the smiling golden sun. As I stepped closer to the open window, I felt an immense affinity with these welcoming rays.

'Don't go,' they seemed to murmur as they caressed my face, 'Stay here – we don't want to shine without you!'

Nature here was already perfect; no surgical touch of mine was needed to improve it. If California desired my company, she certainly had no ulterior motives! She loved people, and in return people could hardly help loving her. Why should I, then, rebuff her hospitality? She was all I had ever dreamed of.

Yes, I would put my signature to this contract I had been offered by Prince's Gate new owners. I would continue with the work to which I had grown so attached, amongst natural, informal people who became one's friends as quickly as did their sun!

To wind up my affairs finally, I decided to write to my family and consult them.

I waited. One day, two days, three – a week. Not a word, not a sign! At the best of times, I was none too good at waiting; I loathed this nerve-racking wait! I asked, therefore, for the two weeks' holiday still owing to me, with the intention of using it for paying a little surprise call on my undecided family. Surely, if our decision was to be truly unanimous, then I too would have to cast my vote into the hat!

London greeted me, or rather snarled at me, in its own unique fashion. No hint of surprise at my sudden return on the frowning, wrinkled brow of its sky. And yet – the feeling inside my breast was warm and pleasing! An inexplicable thrill quickened my pulses as my taxi wove its way through the tangle of Piccadilly's traffic. Was this, after all, my discarded love – not California?

'George! – Daddy! Didn't you – didn't you get our telegram? Gosh, Daddy!' My family's amazement resounded from every corner.

'Telegram?' I asked. 'I certainly didn't! What did it say, anyway, this telegram of yours?' It was good to kiss my wife's cheek again.

'Just that we'd all like to be together,' she told me gently.

'Well, so we are now!' I smiled and embraced her.

And together we remained! Yet whether because now I had returned with renewed vigour from the Californian sun – a storehouse of gold – to brave the stern English climate, or simply because I could not tear myself away from London permanently, I cancelled my appointment in California!

Nothing succeeds like success, they say. And this time it looks as if I really have come home. For how long? Only the future will tell.

Then one fine London morning a card arrived from California to rest on my breakfast tray, together with the Scots Oats and marmalade. The porridge tasted particularly good to me that morning as I read the announcement of an addition to the McCullough clan! Only then did I know for certain that my operation on Sheena McCullough had been as successful in its own way as had the one on her Ian. The 'bairn' was ample proof!

Let us hope, in all sincerity, that my unusual wedding-gifts were a wee contribution, at least, to the nuptial bliss of these Scots-American 'Love Birds'!

XV

An Old Shakespearian Ordeal

There can be no mistake about it. My first patient I saw after my return to London was undoubtedly one of my more successful cases. I accepted long odds against pulling it off, and my faith was justified. Such a case always brings a glow of satisfaction to a doctor. It means another life saved, another human being rescued from suffering, another family and circle of friends from which the grim shadow of impending tragedy has been lifted.

Yet it is for none of those reasons that the case remains so deeply inscribed on my memory. Of course, I like to remember the technical aspect of it. Who does not enjoy reflecting upon a piece of work well done? But it is for the fascinating personality, the almost fantastic atmosphere, that I regard this case as noteworthy and worthy of something more than my own private thoughts and a cold entry in my casebook.

So it is – or should be – with all one's cases. Memories of the people should remain long after the technical details have become dim. The doctor, no matter whether his practice lies in Harley Street or Harrow, whether he be general practitioner or specialist, who allows every newcomer to his consulting room to be no more than 'another case' ends up by being a bad doctor – if he is not already one to start with.

My first introduction to Mr Latimer Whailey was through his daughter, whom I had met informally somewhere or another. She was looking, I remember, worried and depressed. There was something, I could see, weighing heavily on her mind. There was no topic of conversation that could hold her attention for long.

After a little while the shadow came over her face again and her dark thoughts, whatever they might be, oppressed her, occupying her whole attention. I felt sorry for her but there was nothing I could do about it. After all, what greater impertinence is there than to pry into another's private worries, unasked? Besides, one of the earliest lessons I learnt on coming to this country was that the English like to keep their sorrows to themselves and that indiscreet inquiries, however well intentioned, are usually met with that 'Oh, nothing's the matter, really. A bit under the weather, I suppose' – which is the most crushing recommendation to mind one's own business that I know.

I talked to her as best I could, thinking that I might distract her a little and turn those brooding thoughts away from their focus, if only for a moment or two. And as so often happens, she felt my unspoken sympathy and quite suddenly, without warning, began to tell me all about it. She did so diffidently, and I think a natural reluctance to be suspected of cadging for professional advice held her back a little.

'It's a horrible thing,' she said, commenting on her own thoughts, which had no kind of connection with what we had been discussing, 'when you've got to sit back and watch someone you're very fond of die before your eyes.'

I looked at her in some surprise. This glimpse of what was distressing her took me off my guard.

'It is,' I replied, rather unhelpfully. I waited and did not press. If she wished to tell me, it would come of its own accord.

'It's my father,' she said slowly, after a thoughtful pause.

'He is seriously ill?' I asked.

She nodded. "Hopelessly. I have done everything. He has been X-rayed and I suppose there's no escape from it. Cancer, doctor.' She shuddered. It is the disease people fear most. The very word makes the bravest shiver: cancer – the crab whose pitiless claws can so rarely be loosened once they have taken a firm hold. The one thing is to kill the creature as soon as its nippers give the first pinch. 'They say it is inoperable.'

I expressed my sympathy. I wanted to help her. What

doctor does not wish he had a magician's wand when he hears those words – 'inoperable – incurable' uttered in his presence? One feels as though one has been personally indicted in the name of the whole profession, the whole science and art of medicine and surgery.

She told me more about her father.

'He is so resigned,' she said. 'He takes it all so philosophically. But then he has good friends.' She smiled rather sadly.

'Friends are a great blessing,' I returned.

'They are not ordinary human friends,' she explained. 'They were born over three hundred years ago, and they live today – particularly for him. You know, doctor, he is a great Shakespearian. He knows the plays by heart, and I think the characters, great and small, are the only real things in the world for him.'

I opened my eyes a little. I have met all sorts and conditions of men but I have not mixed much with great scholars.

'He is a professor – a lecturer?' I inquired.

She laughed. It was the first time I had seen her amused that day. The dark expression lifted momentarily from her face.

'No,' she said, shaking her head. 'He has no use for these people who tear Shakespeare to pieces, as he puts it. The plays are living things to him. No, Daddy's no professor,' she went on. 'He's nothing at all wonderful. He just keeps a shop – and by the way, it's not so far from your hospital.'

I was interested. A shopkeeper who knew the plays of Shakespeare by heart, who lived in a world peopled by the greatest characters of drama, was certainly a novelty to me. But I could not seek to gratify my curiosity then. It was time for me to go.

I said good-bye to her, murmuring some commonplace hopes that even the best of doctors has been sometimes proven wrong. And in the next few days, in the press of newly-started work, I admit I practically forgot the shopkeeping Shakespearian. After all, daughters, especially those as fond of their fathers as this one was, often magnified their father's abilities; the trick of being able to quote a few lines might well be the factual basis for this legend I had heard ... An ungenerous thought, one of which I am now ashamed, but perhaps not unnatural.

Destiny ordained that I was to meet this scholar of the stores. And the appointed time came soon. I was summoned to see an urgent case, not at the hospital but at his home ... A Mr Latimer Whailey ... I groped in my memory to explain the familiarity this name had for me. Whailey? Oh, yes, of course: the Shakespearian ...

His daughter admitted me to the small, attractive house, She spoke to me quickly, quietly, and seriously. Her father was very, very ill. I had been called in as a last desperate resort. She trusted me. If I said that nothing could be done, then she would accept it as final. And while she talked I let myself unobtrusively take in the atmosphere of the room.

Yes, it was a scholar's room, with shelves filled with Shakespeariana. The plays in many editions, old and new; commentaries; the monographs of theorists and speculators. There were books everywhere, but only on one subject, that which for two centuries and more has provided scholars and pedants, essayists and doctrinaires, with an inexhaustible mine: William Shakespeare, the poet and dramatist whose works are familiar to many, many people and many lands, but whose life and the manner of it remains as obscure as the very cause of genius itself.

But my presence there was not due to an interest in Shakespeare; I was there as a surgeon urgently summoned to a serious case; and I asked to be taken at once to the patient.

He was in bed, and my heart sank as I glanced at his face. It was quiet, almost serene in expression, though perhaps not at all remarkable in its features. On it were the marks that I had come to know only too well, the scorings that are carved by the first tentative graspings of the hand of death.

He smiled at me, and I began my examination. Once more my heart sank. I knew what the X-ray photographs had shown, but this was a case in which X-rays were but a confirmation. Those diagnosticians of past generations, who with their sensitive fingers, their appraising eyes, and clear logical minds, knew nothing of the aids we modern doctors regard as essential, would have had no doubt about this case. It presented no difficulty at all. Below the costal margin was a lump that even the least experienced fingers could detect. It was one of the largest I had ever felt. Yes, it was a desperate case. Inoperable? Yes, of course.

All the time he had lain back in perfect relaxation, offering no comments, concerned, so it seemed, just with the act of breathing. And then his voice came to me, clearly, distinctly, and cut through the dark cloud of thought that wrapped me. It was his voice; but the words were the words of Shakespeare, famous above even the many famous lines of that superb poet with whom England enriched the world: the words of Hamlet: 'To be or not to be ...'

He went on, savouring the words on his palate, like a connoisseur with his Château-Yquem. How many times had he read and quoted those words, I wondered. Yet one could hear that they were ever fresh to him, that every time he recalled them he saw some new beauty in their form, some new profundity in their thought, as a lover sees ever some new enchantment in his mistress.

To be or not to be – that is the question –
Whether 'tis nobler in the mind to suffer
The slings and arrow of outrageous fortune ...

Here, in truth, were the slings and arrows of outrageous fortune! But they were only indirectly of the mind; perhaps not there. For this man had the philosophy of the master in whose steps he followed. One believed he would face death without a qualm, like Hamlet himself.

'Or to take arms against a sea of troubles,' he continued – 'And by opposing end them ...?'

That was my question, not his. Here indeed was a sea of trouble. Had I the arms to oppose them?

'... To die – to sleep –
No more; and by a sleep to say we end
The heartache and the thousand natural shocks
That flesh is heir to ...'

Was he consciously putting his case to me through these immortal words? The alternatives were put plainly before me, with a vividness nothing could have brightened. On the one side, death; on the other vigorous action. And the weariness, the yearning to die – to sleep – was that, too, an expression of his own deep longing? Did he feel that it was time to cry 'Enough!' – and with it perhaps the doubt whether he had the courage for death?

A doctor must order his conduct by the rules of science. But he is also a human being, in whom are the same dark well-springs of thought and action as other men know. Perhaps because his experience of humanity – and particularly suffering humanity – is wider than most men's, he becomes hypersensitive. He has to make bold and big decisions that may mean the saving of a life – or its cessation. Science, the cold logic of the laboratory, has not the answer to all his problems, particularly if he is a surgeon. For to a surgeon the last question is always: Can I do it? His knowledge and experience may tell him that such and such a thing is possible. But beyond that is his own skill and whether it can turn possibility into actuality.

I do not say that it was the magic of Hamlet's words that led me to my decision, but I do say that their coming at that time focused my mind precisely on the questions at issue. Surely this was a case of to be or not to be – and that question could not be left to resolve itself but had to be tackled immediately.

So it was that, in that minute, I determined upon a bold course. Some perhaps may call it foolhardy, but I do not think so. As I saw it there was a ray of hope; and if there is such a ray it is not for the doctor to pull down the blinds; rather he should seek to turn it into a bright gleam that grows. 'Inoperable' is a big word I do not like. It does not mean quite what it says, for it suggests a knowledge – an omnipotence – among the medical profession that those with the widest experience would be the last to claim. What it means in the vast majority of cases is that those who pronounce it do not think they have the skill necessary to do the work in hand – or that our knowledge is so limited that none of us knows the way. And it is that which makes so many dubious about the rightness of euthanasia – but this is digressing from my theme.

There was that chance and I resolved to take it. I would, if the patient and his family consented, open the abdomen and then with the full facts before me decide what could be done.

Had he the courage? I thought so. And I believed, too, that it was my duty to explain to him personally what I proposed to do, exaggerating rather than minimizing the risks, leaving no possible doubt in his mind that the possible – nay the probable – result was death.

For the first time he spoke to me. It was almost as though he had divined my thoughts.

'It's hopeless, doctor?' he asked.

'Not quite as bad as that,' I replied, though in a serious voice. 'I think there is a faint ray of hope, but the risk is enormous and the odds against success are very long. The question is whether you're prepared to take the risk?'

'What does it matter, doctor?' he returned with a resigned air. 'If I am to die, I must die. It makes no difference whether I go now, through trying to fight it, or if I wait till that thing kills me.'

'It is a very serious operation,' I insisted, 'that I propose to make. Almost, but not quite, a counsel of despair.'

He smiled faintly and replied in the words of Shakespeare; it was as though quotation was more habitual to him than ordinary speech.

'Diseases desperate grown,
By desperate appliance are relieved,' he said. *Hamlet* again.

'True. Would you like to talk it over with your daughter? There is not need to make an emergency operation of it, you know.'

'No thanks, doctor. I know she would like me to take the risk, as you put it, though to me all thoughts of risk have gone. When there's a certainty before you, the only thing is choice of means. But I have one request to make.'

'Yes?' I did not quite know what to expect. Patients sometimes make the most curious requests on these occasions, and I am never surprised at what they ask.

'Can it be next week?'

I thought quickly and nodded. 'Yes. I think it can be arranged at the hospital.'

'Thank you. I have a special reason for that,' he explained. 'You see, next week I shall be seventy-five, and if I must die I'd rather die on my birthday. Shakespeare did, so they say, but that's absurd, because he can never die. No, my reason is more practical. I don't want people arguing about my age. So if it's next Thursday, they can say I died on my seventy-fifth birthday, without any months or days. Besides, it would finish off the whole business very tidily, and I've always been a tidy man.'

'Very well.' It was a request I had never had before, but it was typical of the man, concerned not with what he evidently considered the almost certain fact of death but with its seemly occurrence. He had nurtured his mind and soul on the perfection of a poet's creation and he wished his own humble life to be some faint echo of it.

'I shall give you a local anaesthetic,' I said, discussing the necessary details with him. 'It is the better way at your age and state of health. It may take a long time.'

'Yes, I am glad of that. I think I should prefer it like that.'

And so after a little more talk I left him. The words of the Soliloquy were still ringing in my ears. I was embarking on an 'enterprise of great pith and moment' in earnest. Yet I had no doubts. I did not disguise to myself that the chances of success were extremely small; that would have been the height of foolishness. But I was glad that I had made up my mind to seize that small chance to do with it what I might.

His quiet courage in the face of what was almost certain death, his sure mastery of himself, his natural faith: those were things worth making a fight for, worth trying to preserve in a world in which racial hate and violence and death were a daily occurrence.

He already interested me deeply as a person and not simply as a case presenting very special anxieties and problems, and in the few days before he was admitted to the hospital I learnt a little more of him. It was chiefly of his immense Shakespearian knowledge, I had heard him quote one of the most famous of all the familiar passages of Shakespeare. I had heard him make use of two lines from the same play – which incidentally, expressed more picturesquely an aphorism of one of the earliest medical authorites in the world, Hippocrates. By itself that was no test of wide Shakespearian learning. But now I gathered that all the plays were his province, that he was as familiar with the lines and characters of such minor people as Audrey in *As you Like It* as with the cosmic reflections of Hamlet or the symbolic imagery of Prospero. The plays were his life; and I began to feel, in an odd sort of way, that to save his life was to save, too, something of the eternal Shakespearian tradition – a tradition whose force I had first felt personally even through the barriers that translation into Russian and other Slavonic tongues set up. For that is the supreme wizardry of Shakespeare's creations. A master of words, almost the maker of a new language, so did he vitalize English, his characters and thoughts and philosophy shine through even an alien idiom of speech and thought.

There was little opportunity of thinking of Shakespeare, however, when he was brought into the operating theatre. After starting the slow-running blood transfusion through both of his arms' veins, I made the incision, and desperate though I knew the case to be I was perhaps not quite prepared for what was now revealed. The growth was larger than I had any reason to expect, and the whole of the pylorus – the connection between the stomach and the intestine – was involved. The obstruction was complete, and if it had been left, death would not have been long delayed.

For over two hours we worked on that stomach obstruction. The patient was, of course, conscious all the time, though he felt no pain, and I was never more grateful for the gift of local anaesthesia. I doubt if a man of his age and utterly debilitated condition could have withstood a long period of general anaesthesia, and I should have had to work against the clock, which would in all probability have destroyed that one faint chance of success – a chance that looked, now I knew all, even smaller than ever.

For some time, Latimer Whailey, the quiet Shakespearian scholar with the soul of a hero, lay quiet behind the drapes that shield the field of the operation from the sight of the patient when a local anaesthetic is employed. Then, when the very climax of the operation had been reached, I heard his voice. It was the same voice I had heard when I had been called to his house – a voice that was his, yet which also suggested that it came from something deep within his soul, bigger than himself. But this time it was not the tortured perplexities of a Hamlet; it was the bold challenging apostrophe of John of Gaunt – lines that have during the recent past been more often quoted than ever before, and yet, despite that fact, retain all their marvellous lustre, like a gold coin in constant circulation.

> This royal throne of kings, this sceptred isle,
> This earth of majesty, this seat of Mars..
> This other Eden, demi-paradise ...

In that setting, the famous words acquired a new and strange significance. It was John of Gaunt speaking, the outburst of a courageous spirit making an exultant appeal against the degradation that he sees before him.

I have begun the quotation at its most familiar place, but Whailey started it from the beginning; and at the very first line it started in my head, though never to the point of distracting from what I was doing, vivid thoughts.

> ... insatiate cormorant
> Consuming means, soon preys upon itself

– how better to describe this cancer, devouring the very vitals of this man? The words, so far from disturbing me, seemed to heighten my sensibility, so that I saw with a more penetrating eye, thought with a more perceptive mind. Above all I saw again how important it was to save this life ...

They have always been for me the most glorious lines in all Shakespeare. The little highbrows may decry them, spurning their glowing patriotism, shrugging their shoulders because they are hackneyed. But are they not rather the evocation of a spirit than the 'propagandist blather of Imperialism', as I have heard them described? Does a pearl, a diamond, a ruby, become hackneyed, merely because it is often worn and delighted in? And now they have forever for me a deeper significance. They call to mind that strange scene, where amongst all the sterile scientific trappings of the operating theatre, the magic of great art suddenly blossomed forth and gave everything a new purpose.

Was he, I wondered, convinced now that all was vain, that the faint spark of hope had glowed less redly and gone out? I almost thought so, for there was a curious quality of intenseness as he came to the two final lines:

> Ah! would the scandal vanish with my life
> How happy then were my ensuing death.

It might have been so. But on me the words had the effect of increasing my resolve that there must be no ensuing death, that I must give more than I had ever given before to make certain that this man who could beckon to death with the gigantic phrase of blank verse should have the right again to welcome life ...

At last it was over. The final suture was closed. I had done all I could do, used every bit of skill and knowledge I possessed. I had given to his emaciated body three pints of blood to help in his recovery. And what now? It had been a major operation – a very major operation. It had necessarily been a heavy shock to a system that was inevitably weak with age, and that had been still further weakened by this malignant growth. The testing time had yet to come. And perhaps the final outcome lay in his hands, for if his courage failed, if his belief in life vanished, then, do what we might with all the resources of a great hospital, death would probably claim what I had fought so hard to save.

Those post-operative hours and days are always the most anxious time. It is then that the idiosyncrasy of the patient shows itself. Failure sometimes comes during that trying time when success seems assured; and sometimes, more happily, the apparently hopeless stages an almost startling recovery. It is these things which preserve one's proper sense of humility in the presence of that complex thing we call a human being, a thing we analyse and dissect but never quite succeed in understanding.

With Latimer Whailey it was, of necessity, a stern fight, a grim and bitter struggle. He had more blood transfusions, but even then the issue hung in doubt. And then the miracle happened. It was as though he had been a beleaguered city valiantly holding out against the forces of destruction and the siege had been suddenly lifted. From then on, it was still a long struggle, but never again was the outcome in doubt.

Yes, it was one of the cases where the long odds had not proved too heavy, a case which anyone might have been excused for refusing. But I do not claim that it was a masterpiece of skill on my part. The final victory, the recovery, was due to his indomitable spirit, his belief in life; and perhaps the boldness which had inspired me, the determination I had shown to bring him through, had been due to those lines of Shakespeare. For, as I said before, the surgeon is a human being and the limits and possibilities of his powers cannot be marked out with the precision of the properties of a chemical. And his resources are not entirely those with which the textbook and the lecture hall and his own practice provide him.

It was some time after I had ceased attending him and had written him off in my casebook – thought not in my memory – that his daughter came to see me. She was still full of gratitude as she had been at the time when we felt sure of his recovery; and she would not listen to my contentions that the triumph had been in her father's own serene and fearless soul. She persisted in regarding me as a miracle-worker – a role which, with vivid memories of the Russia of my childhood days, I have no ambition to fulfil. But she had not come to give thanks to me again. This time it was business.

'We can never repay you, doctor,' she said earnestly. 'There is no price for life. But there is something we can do – and you have never sent in your bill. Let me know what your fees are – and excuse me for being so blunt.'

I refused her offer point-blank.

'No,' she insisted. 'That isn't right. You have given us one priceless thing. Don't give us any more.'

It was not a case for a fee, and I told her so.

'Listen,' I said. 'This wasn't an ordinary case. It was a very great experience for me. Try and look at it in this way. Your father, through his courage, gave me an opportunity of carrying out an operation such as would very rarely come my way. My debt is to him, and you have none to me. He is a textbook case.'

She smiled. 'That's very tactfully put, doctor, and I appreciate it. But I still think it isn't fair. Let me at least pay some of the expenses. I know I can't hope to pay them all – but something.'

I shook my head. 'No, though I do understand and appreciate your attitude. Your father was admitted under the NHS and all expenses were included for his treatment, Miss Whailey. You said just now you were under a debt you could never repay. I don't agree. But even if it were so, I, too, owe a debt to you which cannot be repaid. So the obligation is mutual and cancels out.'

'So you won't be shifted,' she returned. 'You are still harping on the textbook case, I suppose?'

'No,' I said seriously. 'It is something much greater than that, though that is important. It is that through you I have got to know a very remarkable personality – a man of courage and unconquerable spirit.'

She looked at me and rose to go; and I believe there were tears in her eyes.

Nor was that the end.

One evening I arrived home to find a mysterious package awaiting me. I was expecting nothing, and I could not guess what it might be. Luckily I am not eminent enough to fear the bomb by post which some prominent people have received or those engaged in political struggle. But when I had undone the string and slipped the wrappings away, my eyes almost started from my head.

There was no need to consult the slip to see where this had come from. No other man than Latimer Whailey would have given such a gift, or made so stupendous a gesture of appreciation and thanks. For the first time I held an early

Folio of the Works of William Shakespeare in my hand.

I know that if I sent it to the saleroom, it would bring me an enormous price. I know that many a library would bless me unceasingly if I sent to them on loan. I know that merely to turn its pages would be paradise for a thousand poor scholars.

But it is for none of those things that this Folio ranks among my most treasured possessions. It is the thought behind it, the gesture of a man who could give – and gladly – that which in itself was most precious to him, and which held for him the wisdom of the world.

and I treasure it, too, because of the man himself, the man who could bring from its cold, antique print some of its most wonderful lines and make them live when the very breath of his life was seeping from him.

All that was three years ago. His seventy-eighth birthday was celebrated just when I was starting out to write of this. For me the occasion was marked by an unsigned card with two lines upon it. They needed no signature:

... For, from this instant,
There's nothing serious in mortality.

XVI

The Gossiping Scars

I was in a great hurry to reach Harley Street. In my excitement over the successful operation on Latimer Whailey, the amateur Shakespearian scholar and the tea-party they gave me on his coming home I had quite forgotten that I had patients to see at half-past three. It was four o'clock precisely when I entered my rooms.

Happily my first patient was not a very serious case. She was a lady of forty-five who had been suffering for many years past from she called 'indigestion', but what her doctor diagnosed as a chronic appendicitis. People with chronic appendices are the hardest person in the world to convince of their condition.

'But surely you must be wrong, doctor,' they say, 'I have had this pain for years.'

They say this in such a tone that there is no mistaking what they mean. They imply that after all it is their pain, situated in their body, and who are you – an intruder and, what is still far worse, a surgeon – to tell them that is is appendicitis? Should you insist gently, they will tell you that an aunt of theirs suffered from 'indigestion' for years and it is probably hereditary.

I have even known some cunning patients who kept moving their pains just to confuse me. Anything rather than an operation! But these malingerers have to be tackled in a very careful way. They belong to 'scalpel-fear' tribe.

The sight of a knife makes them blench. They have seen dogs and cats run over and they think it is horrid. They are quite right, but they impose their imaginations on their lives, and imagine that an operation table is little short of the rack of the Inquisitor Torquemada and the surgeon some disciple of his who is merely interested in the patients inside for what he can get out of it. (This does not refer to cheques!)

'So, you have indigestion?' I asked. 'Quite right, you have. All abdominal ills start with "indigestion".' That pleased and puzzled her. 'But,' I added, remembering that I had kept her waiting, 'my apologies for keeping you waiting.'

'Oh, that's all right,' she replied. 'I've had this pain for years and a mere half-hour won't make any difference.'

I agreed. But what I really meant to say was that I was sorry I was late for such an unprofessional reason as private tea-party. I did not tell that to the patient. You must never tell patients about your private life. Surgeons, like ministers of the Church, are not supposed to have them. You are a block of stone, a man of talent, an extractor of malign human parts, and that's all.

But if you aren't able to tell your patients the real reasons for your delay, the patients are able to discuss anything they wish amongst themselves in the waiting-room if they want to.

'So,' said my patient, 'please don't apologize. I had a most interesting half-hour looking at the exotic furniture in your waiting-room. I collect oriental antiques and was very pleased to see a Chinese brish-bowl. Had there not been other patients in the room, I might have run away with it. However, the time went by very quickly as a few of us ladies got chatting about our individual ills. It's amazing how pleasant it is to tell another soul about one's sciatica or indigestion. Common aches seem to cement friendships, don't you think?'

I did think so. As I listened to the story of my patient I remembered the numerous friendships that spring up in doctors' waiting-rooms. They seem to be a most popular place with elderly ladies, almost as popular as a bridge-party.

Friendships are supposed to spring from mutual understanding and sympathy, and what better place can there be for the exercise of these qualities than a doctor's waiting-room?

It is not the experience of common joys, such as one finds on a pleasure cruise, in a threatre, or a swimming pool, it is rather the sharing of suffering and the appreciation of other people's suffering, which has so popularized doctors' waiting-rooms. I am certain that one day an enterprising Harley Street surgeon or physician will have 'at homes' or special 'Mutual Pains' teas in his waiting-room. He will be as careful as a matrimonial agency to see that the right sort of pains and aches and complaints come together.

An appendicitis scar, for instance, has very little sympathy with a hernia scar, and the conversation between the two scars would be comparatively limited and might quite conceivably end in a quarrel. But bring together a couple of serious abdominal scars, and they will get on fine, telling each other their experiences and complaining of the harshness of the clinic matron or the charm of the resident doctor. Broken limbs, too, get on well with each other. Here an exciting climax can be obtained by withholding the cause of the accident and springing a surprise on the listener, who then pretends to be overcome with horror and proceeds to tell you his or her climax.

Plastic surgery scars are more reserved. They are busy telling each other lies about their ages and each one knows very well that both of them consulted the same plastic surgeon. Should they discover this without any unpleasant consequences they will lie about the fees. They will boast that they paid five or six hundred pounds more than each other. I heard an elderly lady turn this to excellent account by saying, 'But, my dear, the surgeon simply wouldn't take much money off me. He said that I looked so positively young that there wouldn't be very much to do!' That same lady had her face lifted on three occasions.

Then, of course, there are the X-ray cronies, who carry their plates about with them to every function as if they were testimonials of good character. 'Here,' they say, producing the negative, 'is my liver. Shocking isn't it?' Or 'What do you think of my femur? Frightful, eh? And only if you were to see my urethra – it would frighten you!' She then shows it and you say that you are frightened and then she goes off to someone else to frighten them.

These people treasure their X-rays like heirlooms. I

sometimes wonder why they don't hang them up in their drawing-rooms, because they do not let the smallest opportunity slip by without showing people their shocking livers, or frightful femurs, or frightening urethras. Tea-time is of course a grand time to watch the X-rayites having a chin-wag over their dark plates whilst they sip China tea and eat toasted scones.

My patient went so far as to say that she was actually sorry when the receptionist called her to my consulting-room. She was having a most interesting and intimate conversation with her newly-found friend. When I evinced some curiosity as to what they found to talk about after such a short acquaintance, I was told politely that it was none of my business. She could not divulge the secret. I was taken aback. What was there, I asked, that could not be told to a doctor? He takes precedence even over a husband.

Then we got to discussing her illness. She divulged that it had taken her five months to gather up sufficient courage to see a surgeon. Her doctor's letter confirmed my suspicion, and when she added that her vicar had said that she had not been looking at all well of late, I did not bother with a lengthy explanation. I confirmed the diagnosis and told the patient that there was nothing else to be done but to operate on her.

To my surprise she seemed to welcome the suggestion. It thrilled her, she said. This was her first operation, and although she had dreaded the thought before, she was quite pleased to have the experience. So that gave the lie to my previous assertion, that all patients are afraid of operations. Some apparently come for the sheer novelty of the thing. To have her gall-bladder removed and be given the stones in a bottle to her for keeps was quite an experience!

Number two patient was called for over the house 'phone. Five minutes passed and no one came. I 'phoned again and asked the receptionist the reason for the delay. She told me that the new-found friends were busy in a conversation. I told her that I would wait for a few more minutes and that if they had not finished their revelations by that time, she was to send me the third patient.

Another five minutes passed, and, just as I expected, my

second patient did not turn up; instead the receptionist ushered in a young man of about twenty-one. To my mild astonishment (I have learnt to be astonished at nothing) he was followed by a whole tribe of relatives. I counted at least six, and I was certain there were a few others who did not wish to embarrass the little standing space there was left and preferred to whisper behind the door.

I looked at the young man who was getting so much attention and asked whether I could be of any assistance. All six relatives said I could be. Take a chair. They offered me my chair and I sat down like a parrot on a perch.

The mother stepped forward and recited her child's virtues. The father said that his son had won silver medals for running and obtained diplomas. One of the aunts testified to his moral character, and everybody else nodded their assent. But nothing was said about the boy's illness. It was, I suppose, up to me to find out what was wrong with him, although it would have been common decency to tell me more about his past illness than about his silver medals and diplomas. But I was well-versed in this sort of scene, when a well-beloved son has to visit a surgeon. I did not pretend to be over-curious. A few polished compliments fell from my lips on the youth's intellectual and sporting prowess.

My professional glance at the youth's anatomy revealed a swelling under the chin. I rose slowly and felt his neck. 'Does it hurt there?' I asked the young man.

'It does,' the boy agreed. The relatives approved of this quick diagnosis. How did I guess? one of the aunts asked with bated breath. The growth, I wanted to say, was big enough and it was easy for me to notice it. But the layman gets a thrill of mystery if the surgeon rattles off a list of Latin names and prods him in a sensitive spot.

'It has been hurting you for long?' I asked. It had. 'Now it gives you palpitations and you have a peculiar choking feeling when you run or climb up stairs.' That was so.

'A cyst of the thyroid gland,' I said calmly. 'A cyst. It means an operation.'

The relatives fell back. The mother sobbed quietly. Mothers always seem to suffer most. The idea of cutting out something from their offspring is terrible to them.

I assured the mother that the operation was not at all dangerous if the growth was taken out in time. But, finding that all I did was wring more tears out of her kind heart, I decided to interest the youngster in the process of the operation itself.

I told him, as all present listened with thrilled attention, that he would be fully conscious during the operation, as I would perform it under a local anaesthetic. This pleased him and his parents immensely and they asked if they could be present and watch the operation. I regretted that that would be impossible as the law forbade it. Both the mother and the two aunts shrugged their shoulders in resignation. The father remained silent.

We spent a pleasant half-hour while I explained to him and his relatives the phsyiological significances of a cyst. I drew them its formation and gave them a rough idea of how it would be excised. I knew my young Italian patient. He was more encouraged by these details than frightened. The element of mystery and fear was taken out of the operation for the patient; But not for his mother. She, together with the relatives, had carefully followed my simple description, but somehow she did not appreciate it. She only begged me to assure her that her son would be well. I did this and turned to answer the hundred and one questions that the relatives and the patient were firing at me. It was a sort of duel to see who got exhausted first. I began by answering their questions simply, but finding that they had overstayed their visit by some quarter of an hour I began to infuse my answers in technicalities, which soon bored them. I acclaimed their yawns and had them ushered out. The operation date was fixed and I shook hands all round.

'Well,' I said to my next patient as she came in (I knew her very well), 'have you finished telling your life story to your newly found friend?'

'I have,' she said. 'I have, but don't think that I'm going to tell you what we've been saying. She told me how curious you were when she came in, but there are a few things which even a surgeon should not know!'

'For instance?'

'Ladies' dresses, hairdressers, arrangements for a coming-out party and plastic operations. But most of all the female patients' ages!'

Epilogue

They all came to see me – some by appointment through their own doctors, some on their own initiative. But most of them had one thing in common. They had been treated or operated on by the accepted methods of orthodox medicine. And many had not benefited from their treatment. All those who came to see me left in varying ways. Some certainly went away disappointed. Others found all they sought. Many of them – to my greatest joy – never went away at all – for they have remained as friends.

Some who hoped to find life found if not death, great disappointment. They are the ones I remember with deep sadness. For one never grows hardened to the fact of unending suffering in one's soul, however cold and indifferent one may hope to appear outwards. Some, sadly, were to discover that even the unorthodox methods I employed did not cure them. However, many did discover the way to a fuller life which they had not dared to hope for. And these cases, while they obviously caused great satisfaction, equally evoke humility at the thought that the powers of the surgeon or physician are so immense. That so much power should rest in human hands, no matter what the methods adopted – is indeed a frightening if also an inspiring thought.

All patients when first they came to see me were merely names. Some had been recommended by acquaintances; others were heralded by letters from those sturdy shocktroops of medicine, the general practitioners who keep the flag of health flying in all the corners of the land. But when that flag had to be lowered to half-mast because there was no imaginable way out, they came against their doctors' advice to seek help. And then they did not long remain mere names. Each had their story to tell; a tale of his or her life which like a portrait, depicts the individual.

These then are their tales that I have set down as best I could in these pages, telling them not with literary flourish but with the simple directness that is appropriate to plain men and women's lives. A doctor's patients – the richest stuff of drama – need no dramatisation. It is only the fantasies and paper figures of the novelist's imagination that need to be tricked out with the finery of resplendent words.

The simple human tale is the most moving of all; and it is the simple human tale of happiness and woe, of fear and hope, that the doctor hears every day in his consulting room.

As I sat writing these stories, I relived all the experiences yet again, marvelling at the richness of human life. I may have transgressed the rules, but in the process I reformed many an old friendship or forged new ones. About some I have wondered, left in mid-air, as it were, for they have passed beyond my ken. With others I had cause to marvel again at how strange are the paths that lead people to lasting friendship.

Let there be no talk of all patients being no more than 'cases' to the doctor. He does not deal in mass-produced toys or bars of soap. Each one who walks into his office brings with them a world of their own, in which life's values are frequently entirely different from those of one's own. It is only in the consulting-room that one realises this fact. And when that room is crowded with patients who have not benefited from orthodox treatment, real-life drama commences and the doctor is like the sculptor who has to account for the success or failure of his piece of creation.

It is for me a profound and stimulating thought, one of which I must always be aware; for it means quite simply that one can never treat two people alike. I hope that in reading these stories and the unusual methods of treatment I adopted, both the lay reader and the medical colleague will find it in his own soul reason to forgive and not condemn the bold way I adopted. They too may experience the same desire to come to the aid of suffering humanity by any means possible – accepted or not – so long as the result is the desired one of cure or alleviation of misery. They, like myself, I am sure, never cease to marvel at this complex life of which we are all so infinitesimal a part.

My final dilemma. I have transgressed and readily acknowledge my crime. What would I do if confronted with similar cases in the future? Would I refuse to treat them or excuse myself and opt out? No. Not I. For I know that no matter how unorthodox the method or how unwise the operation so long as I know deep in my heart that it is the only way to save a patient, I will go ahead, irrespective of the clucking tongues or the raised eye-brows of the men of orthodox medicine.

As long as I am convinced it will do no harm to the patient; will not worsen his or her condition, I will always brave the painful condemnation of colleagues. And so I rest my case.